M000083781

Psychology in the Bathroom

Also by Nick Haslam

INTRODUCTION TO PERSONALITY AND INTELLIGENCE

INTRODUCTION TO THE TAXOMETRIC METHOD: A PRACTICAL GUIDE
(with J. Ruscio & A. Ruscio)

PSYCHOLOGY: FROM INQUIRY TO UNDERSTANDING
(with S. Lilienfeld, S. Lynn, L. Namy, N. Woolf, G. Jamieson & V. Slaughter)

RELATIONAL MODELS THEORY: A CONTEMPORARY OVERVIEW

YEARNING TO BREATHE FREE: SEEKING ASYLUM IN AUSTRALIA
(with D. Lusher)

Psychology in the Bathroom

Nick Haslam
University of Melbourne, Australia

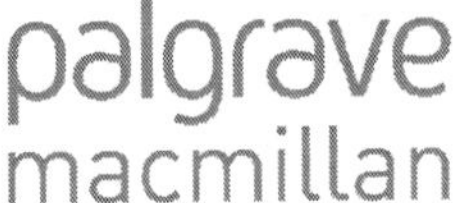

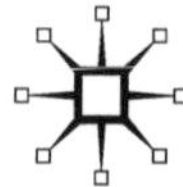

First published 2012 by
PALGRAVE MACMILLAN

Palgrave Macmillan in the UK is an imprint of Macmillan Publishers Limited, registered in England, company number 785998, of Houndmills, Basingstoke, Hampshire RG21 6XS.

Palgrave Macmillan in the US is a division of St Martin's Press LLC, 175 Fifth Avenue, New York, NY 10010.

Palgrave Macmillan is the global academic imprint of the above companies and has companies and representatives throughout the world.

Palgrave® and Macmillan® are registered trademarks in the United States, the United Kingdom, Europe and other countries.

ISBN 978–0–230–36824–8

This book is printed on paper suitable for recycling and made from fully managed and sustained forest sources. Logging, pulping and manufacturing processes are expected to conform to the environmental regulations of the country of origin.

A catalogue record for this book is available from the British Library.

A catalog record for this book is available from the Library of Congress.

10 9 8 7 6 5 4 3 2 1
21 20 19 18 17 16 15 14 13 12

Printed and bound in the United States of America

Contents

Tables

Acknowledgements

Writing a book on the psychology of excretion is guaranteed to pique people's curiosity, but it may not be the best way to garner respect as an academic psychologist. I am fortunate to have received nothing but amused encouragement and advice from my colleagues. Several advice-givers suggested that readers might want to peruse the book during visits to the bathroom and one proposed that its pages might be perforated for that purpose. Many cover designs of questionable taste were put forward. For their support and example I am especially grateful to my social psychology colleagues Jenny Boldero, Cordelia Fine, Cassie Govan, Yoshi Kashima, Simon Laham and Luke Smillie.

Chapter 5 is a substantially edited and expanded version of content which originally appeared in *Review of General Psychology*, volume 15, pp. 351–360. Copyright ©2011 by the American Psychological Association. Adapted with permission. No further reproduction or distribution permitted without written permission from the American Psychological Association.

Olivia Middleton, Melanie Blair, Monica Kendall and the team at Palgrave Macmillan have been exceptional in seeing the merit in an unorthodox project and in steering the book through to completion.

This book is for Vikki, who indulges my desire to write and read obscure texts late into the night and who reminds me that there is more to life than books.

1
Introduction

Philosophy in the Bedroom was published by the notorious Marquis de Sade in 1795. Sade's heroine, the adolescent Eugénie, is introduced to three libertines who alternate bouts of debauchery with lectures on the nature of freedom, morality and religion. Her innocence and ignorance not so much lost as tossed aside, Eugénie becomes a revolutionary who rebels against taboo, social convention and the state.

Psychology in the Bathroom is a different kind of book, switching disciplines and chambers. It is not primarily a study of large, philosophical ideas but an exploration of scientific knowledge about thinking, emotion and behaviour. Its setting is not the boudoir but the smallest room. Rather than studying sex, it examines excretion. This book is an investigation of the ways in which psychological research and theory illuminate elimination and the many phenomena, normal and pathological, that are associated with it.

The psychology of excretion might appear to be an unpromising topic for a book, unsavoury, puerile and trivial. However, it is crucially important and endlessly fascinating. Human waste is an abiding concern for individuals and societies, and our attitudes and reactions to it have implications for our health, our happiness and our environment. Inadequate hygiene and faecally contaminated water cause the deaths of more than two million children each year through diarrhoea and by exacerbating the effects of malnutrition. Faecal transmission is responsible for many debilitating diseases including typhoid, trachoma, schistosomiasis and the intestinal nematode infections that afflict one-third of the world's population (Prüss-Üstün et al., 2008; Rosenquist, 2005). Hundreds of millions of people globally suffer from the shame, discomfort and general misery of gastrointestinal conditions. Billions of people need to be provided with sanitation, water and food in the coming years, and sustainable solutions to these challenges require us to overcome deep-seated attitudes towards excreta. Disgust and contamination fear are the primary sources of resistance to the use of recycled drinking water (Callaghan et al., 2012) and to the use of human excrement for fertilizer in places where chemical alternatives are expensive and food security is tenuous (Mariwah & Drangert, 2011).

Despite its importance, excretion is something that people rarely want to think about. Instead we try to put the greatest possible physical and psychological distance between ourselves and our waste. We prize the technologies we have invented for doing so, even if they are often taken for granted and hidden from view. One survey of the British public's judgements of the most important human inventions found that the flush toilet ranked 9th, one rank above the combustion engine and 73 ranks above Facebook. Toilet paper was ranked 22nd, above trains, pens and shoes. Nappies, ranked 62nd, were adjudged a better thing than sliced bread (70th).

These rankings might seem to inflate the importance of sanitation, but a case can be made that it is an essential foundation for the development of modern societies. The dread of parasite-borne disease, one consequence of deficient sanitation, appears to be a significant basis for prejudice, repression and tribalism. These forms of social exclusion and separation thrive on fears of contagion and the belief that other groups are impure and contaminating. People who are more xenophobic and ethnocentric tend to perceive greater risk of infectious disease (Faulkner et al., 2004) and people living in countries with higher levels of parasite stress tend to be more cautious and less open to new ideas and experiences (Schaller & Murray, 2008). This link between infectious disease threat and intolerance can be understood as a kind of behavioural immune system, guarding us against contagion at the cost of distrust and closed-mindedness. It has even been argued that democratic societies with liberal values and developing economies emerged as a result of reductions in parasite stress, due in part to improvements in sanitation (Thornhill et al., 2009). Indeed, Thornhill and colleagues found that countries with high levels of parasite-borne disease were much less likely than others to have a robust democracy, individual freedom, equitable distribution of economic resources and gender equality.

In addition to having broad societal implications, excretion is psychologically important in a number of ways. As much as people tend to keep them quiet, hidden and deeply private, defecation and urination are universal parts of the human experience. They are also processes that remind us of our animality and our vulnerability to death and decay. Most people engage in these processes more frequently and with less choice in the matter than any other bodily function, with the exception of breathing. Acquiring control over excretion is a major landmark in human development and a matter of anxious concern for children and parents. Anxiety is only one of several intense emotions that excretion and its products evoke, along with disgust and shame. Numerous psychological disorders are associated with disturbed patterns of excretion or disordered relationships with excreta and many medical problems with gastrointestinal or urological symptoms have large psychological components.

Ideas, images and language associated with excretion provided further evidence of its psychological importance. Words referring to excretion, excrement and the responsible parts of our anatomy are key elements of slang, swearing and verbal abuse, rivalling and even outdoing words associated with sex. Scatological elements are common ingredients of jokes and other forms of humour. Just as abuse and scatological humour draw loud attention to human elimination, it is also obscured and minimized by various forms of linguistic delicacy and evasion. Even the word 'bathroom' is euphemistic: one does not go to the bathroom to bathe, nor does one normally go to a restroom simply to rest. Excretion conveys a rich assortment of psychological meanings and the wide circulation of these meanings reveals the depth of people's interest in it.

Besides offering a window onto excretion itself, the bathroom is also a laboratory for studying other fascinating topics. One such topic is the psychology of gender. In most parts of the world men and women use toilets differently, in a way that reflects their anatomical differences: men often stand to urinate whereas women do not. One indirect consequence of this difference in toilet behaviour is that men's and women's public restrooms typically remain separate at a time when few other public spaces are segregated by gender. A further consequence is tension between men and women over bathroom access and etiquette. Inequalities in the provision and design of public restrooms for men and women are one focus for campaigners against sex discrimination, who argue that women should not have to wait longer than men to use restrooms. The 'potty parity' issue (Anthony & Dufresne, 2007) has led to litigation and changes to the required ratios of male and female facilities in building codes. Gender differences in urination-related behaviour also generate tensions in private bathrooms, with disputes over whether men should put the seat down disturbing the domestic peace in many households.

Gender raises its head in many other toilet-related phenomena that will be examined in this book. Girls tend to be toilet-trained earlier than boys. Women are more likely to suffer from irritable bowel syndrome, whereas men are more likely to have pathological fears of urinating in public restrooms. Women tend to be more disgusted by bodily waste products, more censorious of flatulence and more concerned about concealing their toilet smells and sounds. Men are more likely to use scatological language than women and are less offended by it. Women tend to write toilet graffiti that has less sexual and aggressive content than men. Men are less likely to wash their hands after using bathrooms. Women tend to be judged more negatively than men when they violate norms of toilet-related cleanliness and purity. Evidently the bathroom is a place that is intimately bound up with masculinity, femininity and the social codes and expectations that maintain them.

Excretion and psychoanalysis

Excretion has attracted the interest of some of the great psychological theorists. People with only the slightest familiarity with psychology are aware of psychoanalysis and its prurient interest in those bodily functions and anatomical regions that we prefer to keep hidden. They know that Sigmund Freud believed that even small children were sexual beings, whose focus of erotic concern progressed through a series of psychosexual stages, each defined by a mucous membrane, on their precarious way towards adult sexuality. In the oral stage the infant's sensual life centres on the stimulation of its mouth, extracting pleasure as well as milk from the breast. During the anal stage the toddler develops increasing control over its voluntary muscles and in particular learns to control its anal and urethral sphincters in the process of toilet training. According to Freud and his followers, children in this stage enjoy the release and withholding of faeces in a way that is sensual rather than merely the instrumental pleasure of learning a new skill.

Excretion figured not only in the psychoanalysts' accounts of child development, but played a prominent role in other aspects of their theorizing. They argued that certain forms of personality and mental disorder were 'anal' in nature, having their origins in conflicts during early child development. People with personality traits such as stubbornness, rigidity, perfectionism and miserliness were considered to have 'anal characters'. Patients suffering from obsessions – many of which involved feeling dirty and contaminated – and compulsions – which commonly involved cleaning or putting things in inflexible orders – were diagnosed with anal dynamics. Two of Freud's most famous case studies exemplified these dynamics: the 'Wolf man' was dependent on enemas and the 'Rat man' suffered from obsessive thoughts in which pots of rats were attached to the buttocks of his father or his beloved fiancée and bored their way inside.

Urination never received quite the same attention from psychoanalysts as defecation, but the neglect was not total. Freud (1908) speculated on the existence of a distinctive form of 'urethral erotism' – it was associated, he thought, with 'burning' ambition in adulthood – but the urethra never achieved parity with the anus by winning its own psychosexual stage. Freud (1930) also speculated that primal man's resistance of the infantile urge to urinate on fire was a key moment in the capture and exploitation of fire and hence a great step in the rise of human civilization.

Psychoanalysts other than Freud also gave excretion its due. Erik Erikson, who broadened psychoanalytic theory to encompass social development and used it in biographical studies, wrote of the importance of the toilet in the life and work of Martin Luther, founder of Protestant Christianity. Luther was troubled in his early life by anxiety, melancholia, unwanted obscene images and severe doubts about his calling as a monk. Erikson (1958) described how Luther, a man who had suffered lasting constipation and urinary retention, experienced a life-changing theological revelation about the importance of faith while seated on the toilet. In Erikson's view the place where Luther had his revelation was crucial to it, enabling Luther to change 'from a highly restrained and retentive individual into an explosive person; he had found an unexpected release of self-expression' (p. 199). Luther was an enthusiast of anal vulgarity – referring to the Pope as 'fartass' and addressing anal affronts to the devil such as 'lick my posteriors' – and Erikson argues that it was only when he allowed himself to symbolically and literally 'let himself go' that he was able to transform and free up his spiritual life. Later psychoanalytic writers have gone further, seeing anality as a core theme not only in Luther's life, but in the expanding ripples of Protestantism, capitalism and money worship that his ideas set in motion (Brown, 1968).

Excretion may also have had some vivid personal relevance to some psychoanalysts. According to one biographer (Jones, 1964), Freud was plagued by constipation for many years and frequently alluded to his intestinal disorders in letters to friends. He also complained of bladder problems following his encounter with American toilets (Kaplan, 2010). Carl Jung, who split from Freud over what he saw as his overemphasis on carnal motivations, was also no stranger to matters faecal. In his memoir, Jung (1963) recalls how as a schoolboy he experienced a sudden dread while looking upon a cathedral and knew that he must stop thinking about it or he would commit 'the most frightful of sins'. After three days of tormented suppression he gave in and saw God, seated on a golden throne, release 'an enormous turd' onto the cathedral. The young Carl wept with gratitude at this sign that he should not be bowed by the authority of the church. Other psychological thinkers have also been vulnerable to the vagaries of elimination: Charles Darwin suffered mightily from flatulence, and the sexologists Henry Havelock Ellis and Alfred Kinsey both engaged in urethral perversions.

Excretion in psychology

In sharp contrast to the psychoanalysts, modern-day academic and popular psychologists rarely theorize about excretion or refer to it in their autobiographies. Psychoanalysis has suffered an eclipse within academic psychology, its ideas largely shut out of the curriculum and dismissed as pre-scientific and fanciful. Within clinical psychology and psychiatry, psychoanalytic ideas also receive scant recognition, although sanitized versions of some have been incorporated into clinical training and practice in the form of talk therapies.

This eclipse is only partial, psychoanalytic institutes, schools of therapy and practitioners continuing to operate in large numbers, but psychoanalytic ideas have much less currency within mainstream psychology than they did even two decades ago. One consequence of the diminishing voice of psychoanalysis is that discussions of the role of excretion in the human mind and behaviour are scarce.

If excretion has fallen from favour in psychological research and theory, the other end of the alimentary canal has fared much better. Numerous scientific journals are dedicated to the study of eating and drinking, including those that examine appetite and ingestion and those that analyse taste as a chemical sense. Thousands of articles explore the symptoms, causes and treatments of eating disorders such as anorexia nervosa and bulimia nervosa, and many professional journals publish research and theory devoted to understanding and treating them. However, there are no scientific journals in psychology dedicated to the study of elimination and its disorders, and psychologists make few contributions to the professional literatures in gastroenterology and urology, which address excretion from the standpoints of clinical medicine and biological science.

Just as psychology caters to the kitchen while closing the door to the bathroom, it also has a great deal to say about the bedroom. A multitude of psychological journals, monographs and textbooks explore sexual disorders, sexual development, sexual minorities, behavioural factors in sexually transmitted disease and forms of sex therapy. Thousands of research studies report surveys of bedroom behaviour, examinations of the role of sexual satisfaction in close relationships and clinical investigations of people who experience problems with sexual arousal and performance. This scientific fascination with sex stands in sharp contrast to psychology's embarrassed disregard of excretion.

This neglect of excretion cannot be excused by a lack of real world relevance or need. Returning to the comparison with eating, disorders that have lower gastrointestinal or urinary symptoms and a significant psychological dimension are vastly more common than eating disorders, which consume a great deal more media attention. Anorexia nervosa, for example, is a dreadful condition, but irritable bowel syndrome, urinary and faecal incontinence and intense fears of public bathrooms are each many times more prevalent in the general population (e.g., Hoek & van Hoeken, 2003; Saito et al., 2002). Just as everyday people would rather not think about excretion and go to great lengths to conceal evidence of it, psychologists have also neglected and hidden it in their scientific work and theories.

A new psychology of excretion?

Although mainstream psychology may have largely repressed elimination, following the discrediting of psychoanalysis and its excretory preoccupations, the field may now be ready to pay proper (or improper) attention to it. Several trends within psychology make this return of the repressed seem more likely. These include a renewed interest among psychologists in the content of mental life rather than abstract processes; a new interest in emotions that are intimately associated with excretion but that had been ignored until recent years; and an increasing recognition of the extent to which mental and bodily phenomena are interwoven. These developments signal that the time is ripe for psychologists to take a second look at excretion.

The new psychology of life domains

One such development is academic psychology's revived emphasis on everyday domains of behaviour rather than broad psychological processes. As Paul Rozin (2006) has argued, research psychologists have traditionally aimed to understand the mind and behaviour in terms of laws of learning, memory, perception and reasoning rather than examining how people think and behave in particular areas of human activity such as sport, work, music, eating, morality or religion. Their goal has been to discover processes that generalize across domains of activity, rather than exploring the patterns that are specific to each domain. The content of particular life domains has frequently been left to the neighbouring social sciences such as sociology and anthropology, with their focus on institutions, kinship, religion and culture, and they tend to be de-emphasized in psychology's textbooks. Nevertheless, as Rozin observes, large changes are underway and a psychology that takes life domains seriously is on the rise.

Evidence of these changes can be seen in several developments in the field. One is the emergence in cognitive psychology of the idea that many important psychological processes are domain-specific and that the human mind contains a collection of somewhat distinct 'modules' that are specialized for particular tasks, such as language or reasoning about social exchange. Another is the growing interest in cultural psychology, which points to the importance of content over abstract process in its analyses of food and sex taboos, honour codes and so on. Partly as a result there is now an expanding array of scientific journals and professional interest groups for psychologists interested in particular domains of life such as leisure, work, sex, eating, religion, morality, sleep and much more besides.

It is in this context of a psychology that examines the hitherto neglected variety of domains rather than processes that Rozin (2007) advocates the study of holes: underappreciated and understudied topics and problems. One neglected topic that he singles out for attention is the 'hole hole', or the psychology of human orifices, which psychoanalysis studied obsessively but which has been abandoned, Rozin argued, by later psychologists. Needless to say, this book aims to fill the hole hole.

Emotion

Emotion has been an enduring topic for psychologists. Understanding the psychological and biological bases of emotion has always been a focus for research psychologists, and understanding and treating disordered emotion – too much anxiety, anger or sadness, too little happiness, embarrassment or guilt – has always been a focus for clinicians. However, psychologists have not paid equal attention to the vast territory of emotional experience, and some regions have been especially neglected. Two emotional outposts that have only recently begun to receive frequent visits from psychologists are shame and disgust.

Shame and disgust are intimately linked to people's concerns about their bodies, and in particular about the violation of norms to do with the body's cleanliness and purity (Nussbaum, 2004). We feel shame most intensely when our bodies have let us down in a way that compromises our purity or dignity, especially when our failure is exposed for others to see. Guilt, which people feel when they harm others or violate their rights, attaches to specific acts and motivates us to make amends, but shame besmirches the whole self and motivates us to hide away or sink into the ground. Disgust is felt in response to a variety of unpleasant objects, such as bodily products and decaying or dead things, and is also a response to particular kinds of offensive behaviour committed by others. The two emotions not only share a close relationship to bodies, but are also closely related to one another: people feel ashamed when someone is disgusted with them and feel disgusted with others when they behave shamefully (Giner-Sorolla & Espinosa, 2011).

Psychologists only started to pay significant attention to shame in the 1980s, before which it was largely a poor cousin to other unpleasant emotions. A major database of psychology publications records only 16 articles mentioning shame in their title throughout the 1960s and 49 throughout the 1970s, followed by an exponential increase: 234 in the 1980s, 665 in the 1990s and 924 in the 2000s, or roughly one article every four days. This growing fascination with shame comes from the recognition that the emotion is a particularly toxic ingredient of a variety of mental disorders, more closely tied to psychiatric disturbance than guilt and less treatable than anxiety. It has also been shown to play a significant role in violence, addiction and responses to sexual abuse (Tangney & Dearing, 2002).

The rise of disgust scholarship has been even more meteoric. From a single article in the 1960s and none at all in the 1970s, disgust appeared in the title of 16 articles in the 1980s, 60 in the 1990s and 366 in the 2000s. The sharp upswing in publications is largely due to the work of Paul Rozin, Jon Haidt and colleagues, who showed how this emotion evolved from a simple way of signalling rejection of unpalatable food – expressed by the wrinkle-closed nostrils and clench-closed mouth of the disgust face – to a complex response to violations of purity, sacredness and reminders of human animality: an evolution of disgust from 'oral to moral' (Rozin et al., 2009). Other writers have explored the emotion as a key component of an adaptive system dedicated to the avoidance of disease (Curtis et al., 2011; Oaten et al., 2009). Disgust is increasingly being shown to play a key role in a variety of mental disorders, as well as underpinning a range of moral judgements and social prejudices, from obsessive-compulsive disorder to homophobia.

The explosion of interest in shame and disgust among psychologists indicates that the time is ripe for a new, post-Freudian psychology of the bathroom. Both emotions are tightly connected to our unreliable, dirty and incompletely controllable bodies. Both are prototypically evoked in the context of excretion: disgust by contact with the body's waste products and shame by failure to eliminate them in the proper way or in the proper place. It is no accident that Erikson (1963) directly linked shame to the anal stage of development, seeing it as an outcome of parents' authoritarian attempts to usurp the child's capacity to freely govern its own musculature. Psychology's new-found openness to these body-focused emotions makes it an excellent time to explore the psychology of excretion.

Mind/body connections

Growing interest in body-focused emotions is just part of a broader increase in the attention psychologists pay to the body and its links to mental processes. This increase is evident in several important developments within the field. One is the upswing of interest in the psychology of physical health and the contributions that personality, emotion and coping processes make to resistance to and recovery from illness. Health psychology is a vigorous field that takes the clinical practice of psychology out of the ghetto of mental illness and into the wider world of health and well-being. Health psychologists work in a range of applied contexts, working in hospitals and clinics to assist in the treatment and prevention of cancer, heart disease, addiction and neurological conditions.

Part of what health psychology has done is to reveal the close connections between physical and psychological well-being. The intimacy of mind–body connections is hardly news any more, but health psychologists have given them a solid scientific grounding. We now have a deeper appreciation of the ways in which mindsets affect perceptions of pain, personality traits influence longevity and susceptibility to disease, styles of coping promote or impede recovery from illness, and simple interventions that target thinking and feeling can have profound effects upon physical well-being.

Another sign of the increased openness of psychologists to the body is a recent line of research on embodiment (Niedenthal et al., 2005). This work reveals the subtle and sometimes remarkable ways in which everyday psychological processes are linked to the body's movements, postures and expressions. People who read words that subtly prime the stereotype of the elderly subsequently walk more slowly, as an elderly person would (Bargh et al., 1996). People instructed to hold a pen on their upper lip feel sadder than those instructed to hold it between their teeth, unaware that these tasks work their mood magic by configuring their faces into frowns and smiles (Strack et al., 1988). People like unfamiliar designs more if they view them while pushing upward on a table from underneath, a movement that signifies approach, than if they are pushing down on the table, signifying avoidance (Cacioppo et al., 1993). People who are encouraged to mimic the expressions, gaze directions and head orientation of photographed faces remember them better than people who are prevented from mimicking by being asked to chew gum (Zajonc et al., 1982). People made to resist the urge to urinate after consuming a large drink make more self-controlled financial decisions (Tuk et al., 2011).

Findings like these show that perceiving, thinking, feeling and interacting with others do not take place on some ethereal mental plane. Instead, these processes are paralleled, shaped and given metaphorical form by bodies that occupy space, and move and encounter other bodies. All of this work shows that psychology cannot concern itself with pure mind but must take the body seriously. And if we take the body seriously, we have to consider it in all its aspects, beautiful and ugly, proud and shameful, clean and dirty.

An overview of the book

This book contains a series of chapters on an assortment of topics connected to excretion and its psychological dimensions. The chapters are intended to stand alone as distinct essays, although they are all interlinked. My aim in writing them is not to deliver profound observations on the nature of the human mind or to draw broad theoretical conclusions, but simply to review what psychological research and thinking have taught us about the topic at hand. Emphasis falls on the myriad theoretical ideas and empirical findings that have been reported in the psychological literature. These ideas and findings are spread thinly across hundreds of sometimes obscure scientific journals that are accessible only to specialists. Many of the papers in which they appear are old and neglected, rarely read or cited. Nevertheless, these findings often contain fascinating nuggets of empirical truth and theoretical speculation, as well as the occasional historical curiosity or titillating case study. My hope is that by gathering up a dazzling assortment of facts, figures and theoretical figments I can provide a basis for psychological understanding on a neglected topic.

The next three chapters of the book examine the psychology of phenomena that are directly related to excretion in its solid, liquid and gaseous forms. Chapter 2 commences by investigating defecation. In particular, it addresses irritable bowel syndrome, a common condition that has often been thought to have important psychological components. The syndrome involves a variety of unpleasant gastrointestinal symptoms, including constipation, faecal urgency, abdominal pain and diarrhoea, which appear not to have a straightforward physical basis, and it is often observed in people who suffer anxiety and depression. The chapter explores the history of theories and psychological research findings on the syndrome, and draws some conclusions about the manner in which psychological and physical factors combine to produce it. In the process we explore the psychology of constipation, investigating whether it is associated with particular kinds of personality or disturbed thinking, as well as examining the complex ways in which the brain, the visceral nervous system and psychological trauma may combine to disrupt bowel function.

Chapter 3 moves from bowel to bladder. Anxiety plays a significant role in irritable bowel syndrome and it is even more central to bashful bladder syndrome, or 'paruresis'. Many people, and especially men, experience serious inhibitions about urinating in a public toilet or in any situation where their private excretion might be observed. Other forms of urinary retention are not restricted to public bathrooms and more frequently affect women. The chapter explores the origins of these forms of inhibition and the best way to account for the psychosomatic processes that give rise to them. It also examines the opposite problem of disinhibited urination in the form of incontinence and bed-wetting, and the varied approaches to toilet training that have been adopted across the ages and across cultures to combat it. In the process, we ask whether there is any truth to the idea, rooted in clinical folklore, that the triad of childhood bed-wetting, fire-setting and cruelty to animals is an early warning sign of adult criminality. Finally, the chapter addresses the case of people who are erotically attracted to witnessing or otherwise participating in other people's urination.

Chapter 4 explores the surprisingly rich psychology of flatulence, a phenomenon that attracts many uncomfortable emotions, including pathological anxieties and paranoid delusions, but is also a staple of boisterous humour. As we shall see, it has been theorized to serve many functions and claimed to reveal many things about its source, including their personality and musical ability. As with several other topics examined in this book, it also tells us many interesting things about the psychology of gender.

The remaining chapters of the book shift focus away from elimination itself to explore topics that are indirectly associated with it. Chapter 5 explores psychoanalytic ideas about the 'anal character', a personality type that supposedly originates in the young child's attitude towards excretion. Sigmund Freud proposed that children proceed from a developmental stage in which the mouth is the primary zone of bodily pleasure to one in which the anus and defecation take over that role. Children who have difficulties in this stage may develop a particular set of character traits, the so-called anal triad of orderliness, obstinacy and parsimony. We examine the psychoanalytic portrait of the anal character and the empirical research that bears on it. Although that research petered out in the 1970s and is often mentioned only as a bizarre relic in the history of mistaken ideas, reports of its death are exaggerated. Indeed, the anal character has resurfaced under several guises in recent personality research and theory, including work on obsessive-compulsive personality, perfectionism, authoritarianism, disgust-proneness, hoarding and collecting, and Type A personality. Although the evidence suggests that there is nothing literally anal about the anal character, the idea persists in a variety of intriguing lines of psychological inquiry.

Chapter 6 continues the emphasis on matters indirectly related to excretion by investigating its role in language. A large proportion of the swear-words that people use to express violent emotion refer to excreta and the anatomical organs associated with them, as do many of the offensive names people give to those who upset them. This focus on excretion is clearly no accident and neither is the description of offensive language as 'dirty words' or 'potty mouth'. The chapter explores the psychology of swearing and its fascinating cross-cultural variations. Swearing reaches an apex in the psychiatric condition known as Gilles de la Tourette's syndrome, in which uncontrollable swearing is referred to as 'coprolalia' (literally 'shit speech'), as well as in 'telephone scatologia', in which dirty language is controllable but nevertheless compulsive. After examining the clinical literature on these conditions we veer back to the literal from the symbolic by investigating coprophagia (shit eating), a different sort of potty mouth. Coprophagic behaviour is observed in a wide variety of psychiatric conditions and may have a wide variety of psychological dynamics. Children suffering from pica may eat a variety of non-nutritive objects, including faeces, and the activity is also frequent among children and adults with severe retardation and neurological disorders such as dementia. Coprophagia can be observed in severe depression and psychosis, in the context of fetishistic sexuality and even, paradoxically, among people with obsessions involving cleanliness and fears of contamination. This chapter attempts to understand how these diverse pathways all lead to a single, repulsive behaviour.

The book's final two chapters move away from excretion as an activity, bodily function or symbolic resource and address the toilet as a physical location or space. Chapter 7 examines bathrooms as a primary venue for graffiti, specifically a genre that has come to be known as 'latrinalia'. Public bathrooms are ideal hothouses for propagating rude and amusing inscriptions because they afford privacy, allow people to communicate anonymously with others and are associated with activities that make taboo ideas and images highly salient. Psychological studies of the content and form of latrinalia are unexpectedly numerous, and backed by large bodies of research in folklore studies and anthropology. As with flatulence, latrinalia is especially revealing about gender. Because men's and women's bathrooms tend to be segregated they have been seen by some researchers as natural laboratories for studying gender differences in ways of thinking, preoccupations, language use and communication styles.

Like the preceding chapter on latrinalia, our concluding Chapter 8 examines the bathroom as a physical location. However, its attention is drawn to the toilet itself rather than the walls that surround it, and to private rather than public bathrooms. It addresses the vexed question of whether men who share bathrooms with women should put the toilet seat down after urinating. The unwillingness of some men to perform this apparently trivial action generates a great deal of emotional heat, making the issue one of the small but enduring battlefields in the gender wars. The chapter presents an analysis of the comparative efficiency and equity of several strategies for the disposition of the toilet seat that men and women in this predicament might follow. One strategy is the clear winner on all counts, the most efficient and apparently the most fair. However, the chapter goes on to argue that the economic rationality of toilet-seat positioning is not really the point, and that we need a psychological analysis of the dilemma instead. I explore some of the psychological issues involved, and close with some sage advice that might just save a marriage or two.

2
The Irritable Bowel

Classification is the bedrock of science. Physicists classify subatomic particles into bosons, leptons and quarks. Astronomers arrange celestial bodies into planets, stars, asteroids, comets and many-coloured dwarves. Chemistry has its periodic table and biology its taxonomy of living things. Medicine has systems of diagnosis. The science of defecation has the Bristol Stool Form Scale.

Developed by English physicians, the Bristol Scale allows observers to score faeces from 1 to 7 on a dimension of looseness. At the hard end of the scale, 1s are 'separate hard lumps like nuts' and 2s are 'sausage shaped but lumpy'. At the loose end, 7s are 'watery, no solid pieces', 6s are 'fluffy pieces with ragged edges' and 5s are 'soft blobs with clear cut edges'. Stools scoring 3 or 4 – sausages or snakes with or without visible cracks – represent the happy medium: smooth, well formed and easy to pass (O'Donnell et al., 1990). The Bristol Scale has become the dominant method for stool classification, superseding an earlier but somewhat more poetic 8-point scale (e.g., 3: 'Collapsed, original shape still visible'; 8: 'corrugated formations and button-like discs'; Davies et al., 1986).

For all its comic potential, the Bristol Scale has proven to be valuable for doctors who treat gastrointestinal conditions. Scores on the scale reliably indicate the transit time of matter through the gut, longer times producing harder stools. The ends of the scale are particularly important because they point to distinct but interrelated forms of ill health: diarrhoea and constipation.

Diarrhoea and constipation are bodily phenomena and they may have purely physical causes. Infections and caffeine may loosen the bowels, and dietary alterations, lack of fluid intake and long-haul flights can cause constipation. Nevertheless, these intestinal predicaments also have a psychological side. The gastrointestinal system is well known for being sensitive to our emotional state and for reacting to the stresses of everyday life. Intense fear and anger can precipitate episodes of diarrhoea, and constipation often accompanies disturbances of mood and provides a focus for somatic anxieties.

This chapter explores the psychology of these defecatory troubles. The bowel is indeed an irritable organ, sensitive to the vagaries of our emotions in complex and incompletely understood ways. Its sensitivity is due in part to the fact that it has its own nervous system, which constantly communicates back and forth with the brain: top down and (pardon the pun) bottom up. Head and heart stand metaphorically for reason and emotion, but the gut is the seat of emotion much more than the heart, and it influences the brain in fascinating ways.

I begin the chapter with an exploration of the history of psychological thinking about diarrhoea and constipation, emphasizing how psychoanalysts and other early psychosomatic theorists viewed their psychological dimensions. Attention then turns to the modern diagnosis of irritable bowel syndrome, a condition that encompasses diarrhoea, constipation and abdominal pain, and that has a substantial psychosomatic component. In an extended examination of psychological research on the syndrome, we explore the personality traits and psychiatric disorders that are associated with it, the kinds of life experience and stresses that leave people vulnerable to it, the sources of resiliency to it and the ways in which the brain and gut combine to produce it.

The psychology of the bowels

Bowel trouble was a focus of attention for psychologists from the early days of their field. Writing a full century ago, in one of the first books on psychotherapy, for example, Walsh (1912) argued that anxiety plays a major role in constipation. Anxious preoccupation with one's bowel movements can, he suggested, set up a vicious cycle of retention, because 'nature resents too close surveillance of her functions and operations' (p. 269). Excessive worry and concern cause the resentful intestines to go on strike, hampering the forward movement of what Walsh referred to as the 'excrementitious material'.

Anxiety was at the root of a pair of cases of severe constipation reported by Walsh. Two sisters who worked at a mill developed an inhibition about going to the toilet during their long workdays because doing so required them to walk past an office window. Their sensitivity to being recognized as capable of excretion by men working in the office led them to have to accomplish their evacuations on a nightly basis at home. In due course these evacuations became less and less frequent until the sisters were reduced to taking a dose of Epsom salts on Saturday night and spending most of Sunday ridding themselves of the week's shameful accumulation. Nevertheless, Walsh assured his readers that constipation was not always incapacitating, citing a successful French army officer who only emptied his bowels every two months, by artificial means. Following his death at a reasonably ripe age, his large intestine was found to be folded into a large, warehouse-like assortment of 'shelves and pouches' in which the faecal material collected.

Other early writers of popular psychology addressed the topic of faecal retention. Writing on 'the bugaboo of constipation' in their book *Outwitting our nerves*, Jackson and Salisbury (1922) observed that it was chiefly a problem for nervous individuals, in whom a psychological problem was given physical expression. Fearful of their constipation at a time when it was widely believed that the body could be poisoned or 'autointoxicated' by the absorption of dangerous toxins from slow-moving intestinal contents, sufferers' anxieties only made matters worse. As Whorton (2000) demonstrates, the period from 1900 to 1940 witnessed a cultural obsession with constipation, which was held responsible for all manner of ills, including rape and murder, and treated with a fearful array of laxative pills and potions, surgical interventions, diets, enemas and commercial devices. These included porcelain rectal dilators, abdominal massage machines such as the Kolon-Motor and the Internal Fountain Bath. Although these physical treatments might be part of the solution, Jackson and Salisbury urged their readers to relax. A less peaceful path could be risky, as demonstrated by a man who tried to relieve his constipation by inserting a hose attached to a water hydrant, rupturing his colon in the process (Walkling, 1935).

The psychological study of constipation came into its own with the advent of psychoanalysis. According to Freud's classic 1908 paper on 'Character and anal erotism', children during the toddler years – reconceptualized as the 'anal stage' – derive pleasure from their increasing control over their bowels. Viewing their faeces as a valuable commodity and as a potential gift to their parents, they derive pleasure from retaining them. One longer-term outcome of this retentive habit may be a particular kind of compulsive personality style, which we will examine at length in Chapter 5. A more immediate outcome of successful retention may be constipation. Constipation should therefore be observed most commonly among adults with what Freud referred to as 'anal characters', whose personalities are marked by tightness with money and time, as well as with faeces.

Freud knew whereof he spoke, suffering chronically from constipation as a result of a disorder that, according to his biographer, Ernest Jones, was diagnosed variously as colitis, gall bladder inflammation and chronic appendicitis. However, Jones also queried whether Freud's intestinal trouble 'was perhaps also a psychosomatic relic of the neurosis that had so troubled Freud in the days before and during his self analysis' (p. 458).

Freud's views on constipation as an expression of personality traits developed in childhood was for a time the dominant psychoanalytic account. Freud recognized that constipation could also be a manifestation of 'true neurosis', directly traceable to 'excessive masturbation or frequent pollutions [wet dreams]' (Hitschmann, 1921, p. 16). To prevent this condition doctors were advised to warn patients against any form of incomplete sexual expression, at least when taken to extremes, including not only masturbation but also abstinence, coitus interruptus or coitus reservatus (i.e., use of condoms).

Later psychoanalysts continued to pay close attention to constipation, developing a variety of alternative explanations for it and also giving diarrhoea its due. According to these explanations, in addition to being an adult continuation of childhood faecal retention, constipation could also be an expression of a particular kind of emotional attitude, a form of psychological defence, a way of expressing hostile urges, or a physical manifestation of a mental disorder.

The idea that constipation or diarrhoea might be associated with particular kinds of personality was advanced by the Chicago-based, Hungarian-born psychoanalyst Franz Alexander (1934), a pioneer in the study of psychosomatic medicine. Alexander argued that each form of intestinal disturbance is characterized by a distinctive pattern of repressed emotional tendencies. People of the diarrhoeal or colitis type have a repressed desire to give or eliminate whereas the constipated type has a desire to possess and retain, much as Freud had argued. Alexander and Wilson (1936) found support for this view in a study of the dream content of patients in psychoanalysis, finding more themes of giving in the dreams of diarrhoeal patients and more themes of possessing, as well as of attacking other people, in the dreams of the constipated.

In Alexander's view, the constipated personality is not merely retentive but also pessimistic and mistrustful. The resentful logic of their unconscious runs as follows: 'I do not receive anything from others, and therefore I do not need to give; indeed I have to cling to what I possess' (Alexander & Menninger, 1936, p. 541). In the case of a young woman, whose husband was thwarting her desire for a baby, two years without a single unaided bowel movement ended when he brought her a bouquet of flowers for the first time (Alexander, 1952). According to Alexander the same dynamic occurs among people with paranoia: just as they are reluctant to disclose their secrets and strive to be self-contained and independent, so are they loath to part with their unconsciously valued excrement. In a study on this question, Alexander and Menninger (1936) showed that psychiatric patients with delusions of persecution had rates of constipation that were almost three times higher than other patients. Some patients with paranoid schizophrenia directly expressed sentiments consistent with Alexander's view, like one who said 'My bowels never move. I am glad they don't move. I feel stronger when they don't.'

Alexander and Menninger found that depressed or melancholic patients suffered similar rates of constipation as paranoid patients, and other writers expounded on this association. Karl Abraham (1917), an early psychoanalytic theorist of melancholia, believed that it was caused by hostility directed by the affected person at internalized images of loved ones, which the person experienced as self-criticism and guilt. In the case of constipation, the intestinal retention mirrored, in a visceral manner, the retention of these internalized images. A similar idea was put forward by Melitta Sperling (1948), who understood chronic diarrhoea as a 'somatic dramatization' of the person's conflicts with loved ones, complete with a desire to eliminate them in a bodily discharge of emotion: 'If you don't need me, I certainly do not need you. You are valueless to me [faeces] and I am eliminating you instantly [diarrhoea]' (p. 333). Other writers agreed on the fundamentally needy and inadequate quality of the patient with chronic diarrhoea. Groen (1947) believed their attacks often followed experiences of loss of love and humiliation, whereas Dunbar (1947) attributed to them a 'jellyfish personality', excessively dependent on others, unassertive, lonely and troubled by feelings of worthlessness.

Writers on the psychosomatics of elimination proposed that diarrhoea and constipation have distinct psychological signatures. Each has its own set of preoccupations, views of the world and unconscious desires. Grace and Graham (1952) argued that constipated people have a specific attitude of 'grim determination' in which they hold on without hope of immediate improvement, saying things like 'This marriage is never going to be any better but I won't quit.' In contrast, people who are chronically troubled with diarrhoea have an attitude of wanting to get things over with or wishing to dispose of things that extends far beyond the literal zone of the toilet. Thomas Szasz (1951), who followed the same Hungary to Chicago trajectory as Franz Alexander and later acquired notoriety for declaring mental illness to be a myth, took a different view. Constipation, he argued, results from strong unconscious 'oral-incorporative' desires, which might literally involve desires to eat but also symbolically related desires to read or learn. In contrast, diarrhoea results when those strivings diminish, 'usually because of guilt feelings' (p. 114).

These psychoanalytic writers offer a variety of theories on the psychological dynamics of disorderly bowels. In the process they draw a variety of distinctions between the dynamics of constipation and diarrhoea. However, they also make it clear that the mindsets of people with chronic constipation and diarrhoea are similar in many ways. Both groups tend to be neurotic, their emotions as loose or as constricted as their bowels. The constipated may be more pessimistic and depressive and the diarrhoeal more anxious and guilty, but both are miserable.

Irritable bowel syndrome

In more recent times psychologists most often consider disorders of defecation under the rubric of 'irritable bowel syndrome', or IBS for short. IBS is a disorder of elimination in two senses: sufferers experience frequent diarrhoea, constipation, or alternations of both, and to receive the diagnosis a number of alternative medical explanations for their problems must be ruled out. IBS is classified as a 'functional' gastrointestinal disorder precisely because it does not have a known biological cause, such as a specific biochemical or anatomical abnormality.

The diagnostic features of IBS are chronic abdominal pain, discomfort and bloating coupled with chronic constipation, diarrhoea, or both. Pain and discomfort tend to diminish following defecation. Although these symptoms are long-lasting they tend to fluctuate over time, with frequent flare-ups and occasional alterations in the nature of the problematic bowel habit (Rey & Talley, 2009). Constipation-predominant, diarrhoea-predominant and alternating or mixed subtypes are recognized. Together their prevalence in the general population ranges from 2 per cent and 22 per cent depending on the diagnostic criteria in use, with 10 per cent a reasonable estimate. Sufferers are responsible for a significant proportion of visits to family physicians and a large majority of the workload of most gastroenterologists. Dubbed a 'disorder of civilization' (Gwee, 2005), IBS tends to be more prevalent in the developed world. It tends to affect women at higher rates than men, but it can affect people of all ages.

IBS is often found in the company of other conditions. It occurs at elevated rates alongside functional disorders of the other end of the gastrointestinal system, such as dyspepsia (indigestion) and gastroœsophageal reflux disease, a condition of uncontrollable vomiting (Nataskin et al., 2006; Talley et al., 2003). It is also found at above expected rates among people with disorders of entirely different bodily systems. IBS is more common than average among people with the respiratory condition of asthma (Cole et al., 2007) and among women with gynaecological problems such as dysmenorrhoea and dyspareunia (painful periods and intercourse, respectively; Riedl et al., 2008). Symptoms of IBS frequently co-occur with chronic fatigue syndrome and fibromyalgia, a disorder characterized by musculoskeletal pain and tenderness (Robbins et al., 1997). It is probably because of the diversity of their associated symptoms that IBS patients undergo surgeries for non-gastrointestinal problems, such as hysterectomies, more often than other medical patients (Longstreth & Yao, 2004). Indeed, IBS overlaps so extensively with a variety of conditions that lack medically explained causes that it has been proposed as one of a motley assortment of 'functional somatic syndromes' (Kanaan et al., 2007). Evidently IBS has complicated links to conditions that extend far beyond the bowel.

The psychology of IBS

If IBS is associated with numerous medically unexplained physical symptoms, it is reasonable to ask whether it has a psychological component. Patients with IBS are very divided on this issue (Stenner et al., 2000). Some view their condition as a stress-related one that reflects their vulnerable personalities, others as a purely physical illness with no link to traumatic experience, personality or psychological dynamics, and still others see it as a direct consequence of childhood trauma. The same disagreements are commonly observed among people whose difficulties seem to straddle mind and body: some fiercely disavow any psychological contribution to their suffering whereas others accept that possibility and with it the explanatory ambiguity of having a psychosomatic condition. So what is the truth of the matter in the strange case of IBS?

Since the time of the early psychoanalysts it has been noted that people who experience chronic constipation or diarrhoea may have distinctive personalities, psychiatric problems or life circumstances. Let us examine each of these in turn in the light of more recent psychological research.

Personality

Freud and Alexander both proposed that sufferers of gastrointestinal problems have characteristic personality traits and styles. Constipated people might carry to literal extremes the parsimonious, retentive style of Freud's anal character, or have the pessimistic and mistrustful traits that Alexander observed. Diarrhoeal individuals might be yielding jellyfish, unable to assert themselves and prone to excessive guilt and dependence on others. Both groups might have a generally neurotic disposition.

Most research on personality characteristics associated with IBS has drawn attention to just this sort of disposition. 'Neuroticism' has a long history as one of the major dimensions of human personality, representing a general tendency to experience negative emotional states and to be emotionally reactive and unstable. Neurotic individuals tend to interpret unpleasant life events as more threatening and taxing than do other people and they are known to be vulnerable to psychiatric disorders that involve disturbed mood and anxiety, such as depression, eating disorders, phobias, panic disorder and post-traumatic stress disorder.

Evidence for the role of neuroticism in IBS is strong. A number of studies have shown that people with IBS score relatively high on the dimension and that people who score high on the dimension are especially likely to develop IBS. However, although neuroticism is clearly associated with IBS, it is a very broad trait that is neither specific to the condition nor especially informative about what makes the condition distinctive. Additional, finer-grained personality characteristics might also play a role in the disorder. Indeed, there is some evidence that tendencies to interpret distress in bodily rather than psychological ways and to be unassertive and socially inhibited are associated with IBS.

Evidence that IBS is linked to a specific concern about bodily sensations and the tendency to 'somatize' distress – to express and experience unhappiness in bodily ways – comes from several sources. A measure of visceral anxiety, assessing concerns about gastrointestinal symptoms, was more strongly associated with IBS than a measure of neuroticism in one study, which also found that IBS sufferers tend to catastrophize the physical sensations associated with normal anxiety (Hazlett-Stevens et al., 2003). Another study (Nicholl et al., 2008) showed that people who developed IBS within a 15-month period were unusually likely to seek medical attention for their problems, to have high levels of health-related anxiety and to suffer from a diverse assortment of minor physical complaints beforehand. Findings such as these suggest that IBS is not simply a manifestation of general neuroticism, but is instead related specifically to a kind of health-related neuroticism that gives a physical expression to problems in living. The findings also help to explain why IBS so often co-occurs with a diverse assortment of other physical ailments – chronic fatigue syndrome, chronic widespread pain, fibromyalgia – that seem to share with it an intimate connection to health anxiety, reactivity to stress, and chronic somatic complaints (Aggarwal et al., 2006; Robbins et al., 1997).

In addition to its links with neuroticism and the tendency to somatize, IBS also appears to be related to a particular interpersonal style. One study revealed that IBS patients tend to have difficulties with self-assertion and social inhibition: patients tend to have trouble with letting others know what they want and with being firm with them, as well as having difficulty opening up to others, socializing and joining groups (Lackner & Gurtman, 2005). Patients also tend to show high levels of 'self-silencing', suppressing thoughts, feelings and actions that might create friction in their close relationships (Ali et al., 2000). In short, IBS sufferers tend to be overly submissive, a stereotypically feminine pattern of behaviour that could account in part for the higher rate of the condition among women. Interestingly, one of these studies (Lackner & Gurtman, 2005) compared IBS patients who had predominant diarrhoea or constipation, and found that those with diarrhoea tended to be overly self-sacrificing, consistent perhaps with Alexander's view that chronic diarrhoea is associated with excessive giving.

Psychiatric conditions

Franz Alexander reported high rates of constipation in psychiatric patients suffering from paranoid schizophrenia and melancholia, raising the possibility that IBS might also frequently accompany other mental disorders. Large studies have reported that between 40 per cent and 94 per cent of IBS patients meet the criteria for at least one psychiatric disorder, most commonly depression, anxiety disorders including post-traumatic stress disorder and so-called somatoform disorders, in which people report physical symptoms that are not medically explainable (Drossman et al., 2002; Whitehead et al., 2002).

The links between IBS, depression and anxiety are strong, but the nature of these relationships is open to question. Are people who are depressed and anxious vulnerable to developing IBS, or are people who suffer from IBS vulnerable to becoming depressed and anxious? Are the three conditions all manifestations of some common underlying cause, or is IBS simply a masked expression of depression or anxiety, both of which have associated bodily features? These alternatives may all have some merit, but the evidence largely favours the first. Depression and anxiety are distinct from IBS (Robbins et al., 1997) and they often precede its onset. A New Zealand study, for example, found that people who were anxious or depressed at age 18 to 21 had double the risk of developing chronic constipation at age 26 (Howell et al., 2003), and an English study found that anxious and depressed people were especially likely to develop IBS in the following year or so (Nicholl et al., 2008).

Stress and abuse

IBS is known to have a genetic component, but studies of twins suggests that this component is quite modest, explaining only about 20 per cent of the risk for the disorder. By implication, factors in the person's environment and life experience play a more substantial role in the condition. These factors might be of various kinds and might exert their influence in a variety of ways. People's experiences in their families may predispose them to develop the disorder by a learning process, many sufferers having had a parent with the condition (Levy et al., 2001). Stress and adversity may also play a role. The stresses of daily life might exacerbate the symptoms of IBS in the present among people already affected with the condition. Particular life events might trigger the development of these symptoms in the first place among those who are already vulnerable to it. More distant experiences of adversity in early life might contribute to this vulnerability. As we shall see, there is evidence for each of these possibilities.

The symptoms of IBS are prone to fluctuate and these fluctuations tend to parallel the everyday hassles that affect people with the disorder. Levy and colleagues (2006) observed that the severity of gastrointestinal symptoms tracked the level of current stress that IBS patients experienced, increasing as difficulties mounted and abating when they reduced. This finding is entirely consistent with the role of neuroticism in IBS, which primarily reduces well-being by amplifying emotional and physical responses to stressful events rather than directly causing misery by itself. Indeed, people with IBS may report higher levels of distress than others while experiencing equivalent levels of life stress (Levy et al., 1997), indicating that they react more adversely to stress rather than necessarily experiencing greater objective hardship.

The role of stressful life events in triggering IBS, rather than merely influencing its severity, is also well established. Studies have shown that the onset of IBS is frequently preceded by adverse and threatening experiences such as problems at work or in close relationships (Creed et al., 1988), and that people who go on to develop IBS tend to have encountered more than their share of adverse life events immediately beforehand (Nicholl et al., 2008). Once again, we can infer a role for neuroticism here, as people who are more emotionally reactive are more apt to respond in more disturbed ways to events of this sort.

Turning to the possible origins of vulnerability to IBS in childhood experiences, several studies have shown high rates of traumatic experience in adults who suffer from the condition. Sufferers recalled elevated rates of sexual, physical and emotional abuse compared to people with other medical conditions (Ali et al., 2000; Talley et al., 1994, 1995). The presence of severe abuse such as rapes and life-threatening assaults is especially distinctive to IBS patients. Those with histories of abuse tend to have more severe symptoms and although the mechanism through which abuse exerts these destructive effects is unclear it may do so in part by increasing patients' emotional reactivity (Talley et al., 1998). Sexual, physical and emotional abuse are well-established risk factors for a variety of the somatic conditions that frequently accompany IBS, such as chronic fatigue syndrome and fibromyalgia, and they are known to have lasting effects on the victim's neuroendocrine system, which controls levels of hormones implicated in stress response (Heim et al., 2009). In effect, childhood abuse sensitizes the person's neurobiology to stress in adulthood and IBS may be one outcome. Whatever its mechanism, the effects of abuse on IBS are significant and even extend into abuse suffered in adulthood. One study showed that victims of domestic violence experience high rates of IBS, suggesting that abuse not only lays down the foundations for IBS in childhood, but may also bring it about later in life (Perona et al., 2005).

Social support

Just as adversity caused by other people may contribute to the development of IBS, so can the support other people provide reduce its severity. This may be especially true if, as we have seen, people with IBS tend to be interpersonal inhibited and unwilling or unable to assert their wishes and be heard by others. Sure enough, researchers have demonstrated that symptoms of IBS tend to moderate when the patient feels supported by others and tend to increase when they are separated from others (Lackner et al., 2010). The beneficial effects occur because when patients feel supported they perceive less stress in their worlds: support-givers function as stress buffers. IBS may be an intensely personal condition, but it is an intensely interpersonal one as well.

The gut's brains

As we have seen, constipation, diarrhoea and IBS can be located within a dense web of psychological concepts, such as unconscious dynamics, personality traits, psychiatric conditions, somatization, stress and abuse. These concepts must all be grounded in some way in the human nervous system. Our hidden desires, emotions and ways of perceiving life events have their effects on our bowels by way of processes taking place in the brain and its neural and hormonal communication with our gastrointestinal organs. These effects are enormously complex, not least because there is not one nervous system involved but two. The central nervous system, including the brain and the spinal cord, interacts with the 'enteric' nervous system, which innervates the gut and controls processes involved in digestion. Sometimes referred to as the 'second brain', this system engages in a two-way interaction with the brain along what is known as the 'brain-gut axis'. How these nervous systems are implicated in the bowel's irritability exercises researchers in the field of neurogastroenterology.

IBS and the enteric nervous system

The gut's own dedicated nervous system is a reasonable first place to look for evidence of the neural basis of IBS. The sensitivity and pain-proneness of the gut in IBS – known as 'visceral hyperalgesia' – might reflect the reactivity of the enteric nervous system. Indeed, two lines of research support this possibility. The first asks whether people with IBS are unusually sensitive to pain, experiencing it at levels of objective physical stimulation of the gut that would not trouble other people. If this were true, the abdominal pain reported by IBS patients would be due to hypersensitive visceral nerves sending their screaming messages upwards to the brain's pain centres.

For this explanation to be correct people with IBS would have to display a lower threshold for experiencing pain than people without the condition. The standard way of establishing this threshold is by inserting a catheter into the person's rectum and gradually inflating a cylindrical balloon until discomfort or pain is reported. Higher distensions of the balloon imply higher pain thresholds. As expected, several studies of this sort indicate that IBS patients have relatively low thresholds (e.g., Mertz et al., 1995), implying a heightened sensory capacity to detect painful stimulation. This finding that IBS is associated with altered rectal perception suggests that the source of severe abdominal pain in the condition is to be found in the disturbed neurophysiology of the gut itself.

This neurophysiological disturbance may result from the heightened capacity of IBS sufferers to learn pain responses. Low visceral pain thresholds may develop through the process of conditioning, in which pain responses can be learned in a relatively swift and automatic manner. There is evidence that pain can be conditioned in people with IBS in an unusually rapid and lasting way. One study demonstrated that IBS patients reduced their pain thresholds in response to repetitive rectal distension but healthy participants did not (Nozu et al., 2006). There is similar evidence for the swift learning of conditioned responses in other conditions that are associated with IBS, including fibromyalgia and anxiety disorders (Elsenbruch, 2011). Conditioning may produce an enhanced sensitivity to visceral pain in IBS patients, leaving them with an exaggerated response to bodily sensations. Importantly, this conditioning process can occur entirely within the enteric nervous system itself, without the brain being involved.

IBS in the brain

There is ample evidence that IBS involves some abnormalities of the enteric nervous system, both in the perception of pain and in patterns of muscular contraction in the gut (Gunnarsson & Simrén, 2009). However, it is equally clear that the brain also plays a major role. The most striking demonstration of this involvement is the fact that roughly 40 per cent of all IBS sufferers experience relief from their symptoms when they receive a medically inert treatment such as a sugar pill (Enck & Klosterhalfen, 2005). IBS is by no means alone among medical conditions in having a high rate of placebo response, and that response does not imply that the disorder is 'all in the mind'. What it does imply is that the patient's belief that she has received a legitimate treatment is somehow registered in the brain, perhaps as an expectation of imminent health, and transmitted to the bowel, which at least for a while behaves accordingly. The placebo effect, for all its mystery, reveals the possibility of top-down influence of the brain on the gut.

That top-down influence of beliefs, expectations, wishes and perceptions on the gut appears to be quite powerful. It has become increasingly clear that many of the processes that underlie IBS patients' hypersensitivity to visceral pain take place outside the gut. For example, although many patients appear to have altered rectal perception and low visceral pain thresholds, many do not. In fact, many patients may not be unusually sensitive to pain, but simply more prone to report it. In essence, excessive visceral pain in IBS may reflect a brain-based tendency to judge visceral stimuli as painful, rather than a gut-based tendency to sense them more keenly. One study found that IBS patients were similar to healthy controls in their sensitivity to pain stimuli, induced experimentally by rectal balloon distension, but were more likely to report feeling intense pain, especially if they were experiencing emotional distress (Dorn et al., 2007). Pain has a sensory component but also an emotional one that is based on an interpretation of the subjective meaning of the experience. IBS patients may have a tendency to ascribe a catastrophic meaning to bodily sensations in a way that amplifies the pain that they feel and report.

In an effort to understand these processes, some researchers have conducted brain scans of IBS patients while exposing them to abdominal pain. One study induced pain in several patients and several healthy non-IBS controls while they were undergoing function magnetic resonance imaging (Elsenbruch et al., 2010b). The patient group reported higher levels of pain and showed greater activation of brain regions associated with pain perception. (Other studies also find a diminished activation of brain centres involved in the modulation of pain; Elsenbruch et al., 2010b.) However, when the higher levels of depression and anxiety in the patient group were taken into account, the differences in subjective pain and brain activation disappeared. By implication, it is the emotional state of IBS patients that accounts for their heightened sensitivity to visceral pain. Life experiences may contribute in a similar way, as IBS patients with sexual abuse histories also display heightened brain activation to visceral pain (Ringel et al., 2008). Research of this kind suggests that what might seem to be a purely visceral pain experience is in fact strongly influenced by patients' moods, life experiences and ways of interpreting their bodily sensations. These psychological phenomena exert a top-down, brain-to-bowel effect that aggravates abdominal discomfort.

The effects of stress and life experience on sensitivity to visceral pain are in no way restricted to people with IBS. Entirely healthy bowels may respond in exactly the same way. One study (Rosenberger et al., 2009) scanned the brains of healthy women while they were undergoing rectal balloon distension. After the balloon had been inserted, but prior to its inflation, the women were informed that they had to prepare a five-minute speech to be delivered several minutes later to a group of white-coated 'experts'. One minute into her speech each woman was interrupted, told she had to be scanned immediately and would have to resume the speech afterwards and underwent the scan following balloon distension. This method of inducing anxiety was highly effective and produced greater activation of visceral pain regions in the brain than when the same women were scanned under less stressful circumstances. Just as this acute stress exacerbated the experience of visceral pain, so did more chronic stress: women who reported more ongoing stressful life circumstances also showed a greater brain response to visceral pain than women whose lives were more placid.

IBS may be linked not only to the functioning of the brain, such as its patterns of activation under stress, but also to its structure. Patients with the condition have been found to have an enlarged hypothalamus, a brain structure that is intimately involved in emotion and responses to stress (Blankstein et al., 2010). They also show a thinning of neurons in brain areas that are implicated in the cognitive control of pain, which might account for the tendency for IBS patients to catastrophize and fail to modulate the visceral pain that they are experiencing. The brain is as much a part of IBS as the gut and it manifests the disorder in its changing physical structure.

Conclusions

It would be a mistake to conclude that IBS is first and foremost a psychological condition. This complex syndrome has many aspects that do not directly implicate mind and brain. It sometimes develops after people have suffered a gastrointestinal infection and may be associated with elevated levels of intestinal bacteria. It has an immune component which may result in the gut having a chronic low-level inflammation. It may in some cases be related to intolerance of certain foods. All the same, we have seen how psychology and the bowel are inextricably linked, and how IBS offers a fascinating view of the intimacy of mind–body connections.

A complete account of the psychology of chronic constipation and diarrhoea has yet to be developed, but it would have to look something like this. People with a neurotic temperament – a personality trait that has a substantial genetic component – tend to develop strong emotional reactions to stress and interpersonal inhibitions that leave them vulnerable to depression and anxiety disorders. These tendencies may be exacerbated if the person suffers adverse early life events, such as physical and sexual abuse. Adversities such as these sensitize the body's stress response and leave the person preoccupied with physical sensations and pain, and prone to place catastrophic interpretations on them. This exaggerated reactivity to stress and sensitivity to physical sensation affects many systems of the body and results in a diverse assortment of functional somatic conditions, IBS among them. The tight, two-way connections between the enteric nervous system and the brain make it likely that the bowels will be implicated in this cascade of stress reactions, with the viscera sending heightened pain messages to the brain, and the brain amplifying rather than dampening them. Over time, the brain may undergo structural changes as a result, enlarging structures that orchestrate the stress response and shrinking those that are incapable of moderating it.

Much of this account can be given flesh in the case study of a young woman with IBS that was reported by Drossman et al. (2003). As a girl she suffered severe constipation and abdominal pain, which began after years of sexual abuse by a family friend. As an adult she developed two anxiety disorders and suffered physical ill health. She had a troubled relationship with her husband, who abused her sexually and emotionally, and she felt unable to assert herself with him. Her childhood bowel troubles returned, switched now from constipation to diarrhoea, and became worse as her relationship deteriorated. After commencing divorce proceedings her depression, anxiety and catastrophizing diminished and her diarrhoea and pain almost completely disappeared. Prior to her improvement she rated the painfulness of a medium rectal distension as unbearably severe, and brain scanning showed strong activations in regions involved in the processing of visceral sensations. When this procedure was repeated following her recovery she rated the same distension as only moderately painful and the brain activation of the same regions was markedly diminished. A more striking correlation of mind, mood, brain and body is hard to imagine.

Our intestines are not just meaty drainpipes through which our waste flows. They are emotional organs whose nerves communicate with the brain and respond to what it thinks, desires and perceives. The bowel is irritable, and not only among the unfortunate minority who suffer from IBS. Our emotions and stresses affect it directly, our personalities are manifest in its habits, and the early experiences that help to shape those personalities also shape its behaviour throughout our lives.

3
The Nervous Bladder

Urination serves many functions among mammals. The lowly rat, for example, leaves urine-marks to label its habitat, defend its territory, assert its dominance and advertise its sexual availability (Birke & Sadler, 1984). Rats urine-mark preferred foods and, in what seems a cruel prank, but probably is not, they crawl over their fellows and leave small wet patches as souvenirs. By smelling urine markings rats can detect the sex, age, receptiveness, social status and stress levels of the marker and can navigate in the dark along established scuttling routes. These complexities are absent from human urination, which serves the single function of voiding the wastes that our kidneys have filtered from our bloodstream.

Although human urination is disappointingly one-dimensional in its biological function, it is not lacking in psychological complexity. The child's acquisition of voluntary bladder control can be a focus of emotional anguish and struggle. Adults can experience a variety of related inhibitions, control failures and fetishistic attachments. These phenomena have received only scattered attention within the field of psychology. They nevertheless reveal urination as a profoundly nervous activity, one that is infused with shame and vulnerable to disruption by anxiety.

Early psychologists had little to say about urination. Among the psychoanalysts it took a backseat to defecation. The anus was given its own psychosexual stage and its own character type, but the urethra was not. Some analysts speculated on the existence of urethral erotism and identified the character trait of 'burning ambition' as one of its products, along with a predilection for playing or working with water (Hitschmann, 1923). One writer saw a baseball pitcher's passion for throwing curve-balls as a sublimation of boyhood peeing contests (Frink, 1923). Freud (1932) himself speculated that renunciating the 'homosexually tinged' desire to extinguish fire by a stream of urine was needed for humans to tame flame and was thus an important step on the road to civilization. Despite these early speculations, later academic and applied psychology has bypassed the bladder. In the meantime, significant advances have been made in understanding urination's neural basis.

Urination and the nervous system

Researchers have established that the neural control of urination, or 'micturition' as it is more scientifically known, is far from the simple reflex we might naively imagine it to be. It implicates a web of pathways involving the smooth muscles of the bladder and the urethral sphincter, the striated muscles of the pelvic floor, the spinal cord, specialized structures in the brain-stem including the 'pontine micturition centre' (PMC) and the 'periaqueductal grey' (PAG), and an assortment of brain regions, including parts of the limbic system that are intimately associated with emotion. At a neural level the micturition system is unusual for its complexity and for involving a combination of voluntary and involuntary mechanisms, making it one arena in which desperate urges and strong inhibitions come into conflict.

Micturition is a complex switch-like process. The act of urination itself is triggered by the PMC, which coordinates the contraction of the bladder's detrusor muscle and relaxes the urethral sphincter. This trigger is in turn controlled by the PAG, which monitors the filling of the bladder and also receives inputs from areas of the brain involved in sex and sleep, which inhibit its activation. The PAG is closely linked to cortical regions, sending information about bladder distension to the insular cortex, which registers somatic sensations, and receiving information about the safety of the environment and social appropriateness of urination from the frontal lobes and limbic system, especially in the right hemisphere. This upstream information, which may warn of threat, embarrassment and social ostracism, combines with information about bladder fullness to influence the PAG's decisions about triggering the PMC. All the while a 'continence centre' that neighbours the PMC promotes 'guarding reflexes' that contract the pelvic floor during urine storage and relax during voiding (Benarroch, 2010; Fowler et al., 2008; Holstege, 2005).

The role of the brain in the control of micturition has been demonstrated by neuroimaging studies. In these studies, people with normal or disturbed urinary function submit to having their bladders filled by catheter and sometimes also must urinate while lying horizontal in the brain scanner. Research of this nature reveals widespread brain activation during bladder distension and during the act of urination. For example, one study found that bladder filling was associated with heightened activation in many brain regions. However, among people with poor bladder control there was relatively weak activation of the orbitofrontal cortex, a region associated with decision-making, planning and the weighing of rewards and punishments (Griffiths et al., 2005). Bladder fullness also generates exaggerated brain responses in regions that are implicated in the monitoring of conflict and the perception of pain (anterior cingulate and insular cortex), implying an accentuated discomfort reaction (Griffiths & Tadic, 2008). Voiding is associated with another set of brain activations that enable deliberate action and the control of voluntary muscles (Nour et al., 2005). Subjectively the act of urinating may feel like a relaxing release, but at a neural level it is a coordinated buzz of electrochemical activity.

The complex mechanisms that orchestrate micturition can go wrong in a variety of ways. People may have difficulty urinating in particular situations or suffer from a more extreme and generalized inhibition. Other people may be insufficiently inhibited, urinating when and where they would prefer not to. Still others take an uncommon pleasure in urine and urination, experiencing attraction where most of their peers feel only aversion. We now turn to several forms of psychological difficulty associated with these varied inhibitions, failures of self-control and perversions.

Urinary inhibition

Studies of inhibited urination have generally been undertaken in the clinic, but one of the first and certainly the most controversial was carried out in a natural setting. The evocatively named Dennis

Middlemist and his colleagues (1976) asked whether the proximity of others in a male urinal might interfere with efforts to urinate. Other researchers had shown that people experience stress when others enter their invisible zone of private space and find these invasions unpleasant and emotionally arousing. Middlemist's group inferred that this stress would inhibit relaxation of the urethral sphincter and increase contraction of the bladder. Stressed people should consequently take longer to begin urinating and should urinate for less time. In the first of two studies, a researcher stationed himself at the sink of a public restroom with two banks of five urinals, pretending to groom himself. With the aid of a stopwatch, furtive glances in the mirror and the sounds of urine hitting water, he recorded the time from unzipping to flow onset and from onset to completion, as well as the number of unoccupied urinals separating the person from his nearest peer. Men separated by a single empty urinal took 7.9 seconds to start and then 19.0 seconds to finish. Those with a three-urinal separation started in a mere 5.7 seconds and continued for a leisurely 32.0.

The researchers conducted a second study in a public bathroom with a single bank of three urinals. Entrants to the bathroom were randomly assigned to one of three study conditions, all of which led them to use the leftmost urinal. In the control condition signs declared the middle and right urinals to be off-limits. In the 'moderate' condition a sign was placed on the middle urinal and an assistant of the researchers was stationed at the right urinal, appearing to use it. In the 'close' condition the sign was placed on the right urinal and the assistant in the middle, adjacent to the unwitting participant. Another assistant hiding behind the urinals in a toilet stall timed proceedings, aided by a periscope embedded in a stack of books on the toilet floor that targeted the participant's urine stream. Having a person nearby increased micturition delay (from 4.9 seconds in the control condition to 8.4 in the close condition) and decreased persistence (from 24.8 seconds to 17.4 seconds). Not surprisingly, this research was immediately denounced by ethicists for assaulting human dignity, and critics worried – unnecessarily, it turned out – that it would stimulate 'a veritable flood of bathroom research' (Koocher, 1977, p. 121).

One thing that remains unclear about Middlemist and colleagues' work is how much it relates to bathroom behaviour specifically rather than to invasions of personal space in general. Excretion is usually a private act that involves taboo body parts and functions, so we might expect it to generate an especially high level of anxiety, emotional arousal and inhibition. Men standing shoulder to shoulder at a public urinal may feel not just that their space has been invaded but also that their manhood is being evaluated: others are not simply close by, but are also looking and, perhaps, comparing. On the other hand, similar space-invasion phenomena occur outside bathrooms. In one study, researchers examined stress levels among train commuters during morning rush hour and investigated how it varied depending on the number of fellow commuters sharing their row of seats (Evans & Wener, 2007). Commuters who had more people in their immediate vicinity had higher levels of a stress hormone in their saliva, lower mood and less persistence on a concentration task, a result that was not explained by being in a busier carriage. Urinating may be an intimate private act but sitting down is not, so the micturition delay of Middlemist's participants may have nothing specifically to do with excretion.

Paruresis

Inhibited urination in public bathrooms may normally be due to proximity and space invasion, not excretion-related concerns, but something more is going on for people who suffer from extreme anxiety at the mere idea of using public bathrooms. These individuals are colloquially said to have 'shy bladder' or 'bashful bladder', but 'paruresis' is the preferred clinical term (Williams & Degenhardt, 1954). People with paruresis experience a severe inhibition about using public bathrooms and in extreme cases they may be unable to use the private bathrooms of friends or family members, or even in their own homes. Sufferers commonly report going without liquids, avoiding social events, foregoing travel and having to plan and map their excretions well in advance. In some cases they remain housebound. When left with no alternative but to use a public facility they may wait hours until all urinals are empty or a stall is free and suffer humiliating delays. One sufferer blacked out and crashed to the tiles from the effort involved (McCracken & Larkin, 1991). Paruretics tend not to tell friends and family about their affliction, unwillingness to disclose being one of the hallmarks of shame, and they rarely seek medical help (Vythilingum et al., 2002).

Although paruresis is sometimes described as a fear of urinating in public restrooms, it is not just a simple emotion in a single context. In some cases there is little if any subjective fear, merely a stubborn inability. The dread may not relate to the context itself, or even to the mere presence or proximity of other people in it, but to the possibility of being observed by them. The anxiety may also relate not just to being observed, but to being observed by familiar people or to making others wait. Like agoraphobia – literally 'fear of the market-place' – which is not in fact a fear of a particular setting but a fear of what might happen if one panics and cannot reach safety in such a setting, paruresis is less a fear of public bathrooms than a fear of what might happen if others witness one's attempts at excretion.

Researchers have helped to piece together some descriptive facts about the condition. Depending on the criteria used to define paruresis its prevalence ranges from about 2 per cent of the population to as much as 30 per cent. It appears to be somewhat more common among men than women, making it highly unusual among forms of social anxiety (Turk et al., 1998). Male sufferers tend to be more bothered by the possibility of being seen by other people whereas women are more troubled by the thought of being heard (Rees & Leach, 1975). The condition tends to develop in late childhood or early adolescence and it is often long-lasting.

Paruresis represents something of a diagnostic puzzle. On the one hand it resembles many of the symptoms of social anxiety disorder, such as fears of public speaking, eating, sweating, blushing or vomiting, all of which represent apprehensions about one's uncontrollable bodily reactions being judged negatively by others. Indeed, social anxiety disorder is the disorder that most commonly coexists with paruresis, with depression a close second. However, social anxiety disorder is only present among a small minority of paruretics (Hammelstein & Soifer, 2006). Fear of public urination also lacks a close empirical association with other social anxiety symptoms (Heimberg et al., 1993), implying that it is somewhat unique. Whereas one writer has suggested naming it as one of a small number of 'sphincteric phobias' (Marks, 1987), alongside fears of urinating too freely, others propose that it should be a stand-alone diagnosis in its own right.

The psychological underpinnings of paruresis remain incompletely understood. Paruretics tend to have relatively high levels of social anxiety, in relation to both public performance and general interpersonal unease and discomfort, and they have elevated fears of being negatively evaluated by others (Malouff & Lanyon, 1985). In some cases they trace the source of their troubles to public teasing or ridicule in bathroom settings. They tend to have elevated body shyness (Gruber & Shupe, 1982), but they do not report unusually high levels of sexual anxiety, implying that bathroom dreads are not somehow linked to bedroom insecurities. Although people with paruresis may have exaggerated privacy concerns there is no evidence that they tend to come from small families or communities with low population density. They do not differ from others in education or social class (Hammelstein et al., 2005).

These research findings help to clarify the processes that give rise to paruresis and clarify what it is. People who are socially apprehensive and prone to bodily shame will tend to have trouble in any situation where they might be judged by others. In public bathrooms this scrutiny, real or imagined, may cause urinary hesitancy by adding performance concerns to the emotional arousal that people normally feel in this setting, as Middlemist and colleagues showed. These concerns may be highly exaggerated among some paruretics, involving almost paranoid beliefs about what others are making of one's urinary failures. As with other forms of anxiety, signs of failure tend to cascade, even while the urine stream does not: delayed urination adds to the performance anxiety, heightens self-consciousness, produces counterproductive efforts to will a stream into existence and leads to a self-fulfilling anticipation of failure on future attempts. If the person gives up and leaves before urinating, the relief that ensues reinforces their tendency to steer clear of public facilities in future, creating a learned avoidance (Boschen, 2008).

Treatment of paruresis usually involves some form of behavioural therapy that targets these processes. Sufferers are progressively exposed to a hierarchy of increasingly threatening urination scenarios – from relieving oneself in an enclosed stall in an unoccupied bathroom to doing so while shoulder-to-shoulder at a bank of urinals – usually with the aid of relaxation exercises. Paruretics may also be taught ways of challenging the self-defeating and self-desiccating thoughts that magnify their anxiety and self-consciousness. One therapist gave a difficult patient the 'paradoxical' instruction to carry out all the actions associated with urination at a public bathroom but forbade him to urinate. When the performance anxiety was lifted in this manner the torrent was released (Ascher, 1979). In contrast, medication has had disappointing results, one trial finding that an otherwise promising drug had urinary hesitancy as a side effect, compounding the problem, and another trialled medication led to painfully prolonged erections (Hatterer et al., 1990).

Psychogenic urinary retention

Paruresis is a form of urinary inhibition that is specific to public settings. Another condition with which it is sometimes confused involves a generalized inhibition that does not appear to be tied to particular situations or related to the dread of public scrutiny. 'Psychogenic urinary retention' is a rare condition that is more often found among women, just as paruresis tends to be somewhat more common among men. Urinary retention can have a number of medical causes, but when these can be eliminated the symptom is usually understood as a form of 'conversion', in which a psychological problem or conflict finds expression in a physical symptom. In the current diagnostic system, urinary retention is listed among several 'pseudoneurological' symptoms – symptoms that mimic those due to organic brain diseases or lesions – such as difficulty swallowing, double vision, loss of the sensation of touch and localized paralysis or muscle weakness (Bilanakis, 2006).

Conversion is one facet of what used to be known as hysteria, the crucible in which psychoanalysis was forged, and it is therefore unsurprising that psychoanalytic thinkers were the first to describe and investigate psychogenic urinary retention. Cases of the condition have been presented in papers dating back to the 1950s and beyond. They almost invariably described women who had a chronic inability to urinate that required catheterization. A variety of causes were proposed, many invoking a sexual dynamic. The symptom itself was traced to a desire to avoid penetration, fears of sexual attack, unconscious anger at a sexually abusive stepfather, anxieties over death through combat or illness, guilt over sexual thoughts or actions, or a desire for physical punishment (Bird, 1980; Wahl & Golden, 1963; Williams & Johnson, 1956).

An illustrative case was presented by Chapman (1959). When this young woman was an infant her mother died during a hospitalization. As a little girl, her relatives frequently reminded her that she failed to live up to her mother's angelic example and that her mother might not have died had she not recently been pregnant. Resentful for being made to feel deficient and responsible for her mother's death, the girl developed florid fantasies of competing successfully against her mother and of her mother being tortured by her relatives. She also developed the conviction that her life would recapitulate her mother's. Aged 8 or 9, when taken by her relatives to her sainted mother's grave, she felt a strong and scornful desire to urinate on it. Recurring deaths of her relatives throughout her childhood led her to fantasize that her own life depended on them sacrificing their lives for her and also led her to develop an intense fear of hospitals. Her first episode of urinary retention began during a hospitalization for minor surgery as a young adult, and her second occurred during a hospitalization for pneumonia, not long after giving birth to her first child. Psychotherapy uncovered the patient's feeling that the retention was punishment for her aggressive fantasies towards her mother and revealed how the symptom was meaningfully linked to the urinary content of those fantasies.

Unlike this case, most psychoanalytic reports of psychogenic urinary retention place sexual causes and conflicts very much in the foreground. Whether or not the details of these sexual explanations are persuasive, the recent research literature at least partially supports the analysts' focus on sexuality. It is increasingly clear that experiences of sexual abuse substantially increase the likelihood of urinary retention and other bladder-control problems among women. Davila and colleagues (2003), for instance, found markedly higher rates of urinary retention as well as incontinence and voiding dysfunction among abuse survivors than among normal controls. This abuse need not be buried in childhood repression, as the psychoanalysts believed, to have impacts on urinary difficulties. One study found that Mexican-American women who had experienced sexual or physical abuse from an intimate partner in the previous year were more likely than those who had not to suffer from an assortment of gastrointestinal, cardiopulmonary, neurological, sexual and reproductive symptoms (Lown & Vega, 2001). Urinary retention was the symptom most strongly linked to intimate partner violence, affecting abused women at a 12 times higher rate than their unabused peers.

Findings such as these contribute to a growing recognition that urological symptoms are strongly associated with abuse and adversity. The abuse need not be sexual, it can have effects on both women and men, and symptoms beyond urinary retention are implicated. For example, Link et al. (2007) found that sexual, physical and emotional abuse were all strongly associated with a variety of urinary problems in a random, community-based sample of 5506 male and female Bostonians. Work such as this shows that there is a psychological nexus between trauma and bladder problems, probably mediated by neuroendocrine processes, and that this nexus is a causal one.

Incontinence

Paruresis and psychogenic urinary retention are conditions in which micturition is pathologically inhibited. At the opposite extreme we find conditions in which it is not inhibited enough. These are collectively referred to as 'incontinence' and take a variety of forms. Urge incontinence, which is especially common among women and the elderly, is caused by inappropriate contractions of the bladder, which produce sudden, powerful urges to urinate and leakage. Stress incontinence, which is also more common among women, is produced by increases in abdominal pressure, such as those caused by laughing, coughing, sneezing or exercise, and reflects weakness in the muscles of the pelvic floor. Enuresis is daytime or night-time wetting by children of an age at which complete bladder control would be expected, usually defined as about 6. All of these forms of incontinence bring embarrassment and shame to the person and sometimes disgust to others. If dirt is matter out of place, as Mary Douglas (1966) observed, then incontinence is doubly dirty: body waste where it does not belong.

'Incontinence' has not always referred merely to the inability to excrete in appropriate places. It is the usual translation of the concept of *akrasia* in Aristotle's moral philosophy, which represents a form of moral weakness in which people lack the capacity to overcome their passions and follow reason. Unlike the vicious or intemperate person, who deliberately chooses to act badly, the incontinent person chooses to act virtuously but is undone by temptation. Incontinence is therefore weakness of will, not mere weakness of sphincter. Urinary and faecal incontinence are nevertheless sometimes seen as paradigm cases of deficient self-control. Parents may worry that toilet training has wider ramifications for their child's ability to delay gratification.

The idea that urinary continence is associated with self-control beyond the bathroom may not be far-fetched. Research by Mirjam Tuk and colleagues (2011) showed that adults made to inhibit urgent desires to urinate – after drinking five cups of water as part of a bogus taste test – were better able to resist impulses in unrelated areas, such as not making short-sighted monetary decisions. Even subtle reminders of the need for urinary control – having to identify words like 'urination', 'bladder' and 'toilet' in a matrix of letters – were enough to make experimental participants resist impatient choices. People who identified these words felt greater pressure to urinate and thus exerted greater self-control on their bladders and their wallets. This 'inhibitory spillover' effect suggests that bladder control is not merely an example of general self-restraint, but something that is dynamically linked to it.

Toilet training and enuresis

Adults sometimes forget that continence is a major developmental achievement. At the start of life we excrete promiscuously, with no thought for time or place. It is only later that we learn where we should urinate and defecate, develop the ability to hold on and acquire our culture's toileting repertoire. This learning process represents a gradual and sometimes fragile triumph of voluntary control over reflex, and it is actively and often anxiously overseen by adults. The civilizing nature of their role is captured well in Selma Fraiberg's (1959) words: 'The missionaries have arrived. They come bearing culture to the joyful savage... promoting the hygiene and etiquette of potty chairs and toilets' (p. 59). The savage is not always easily converted and often rebels, and there is sometimes a sense of threat behind the zeal of the missionaries. One study found that a majority of cases of fatal child abuse involving children older than 12 months were associated with bladder or bowel accidents or nappy changes (Krugman, 1984).

The way in which continence is trained has undergone substantial changes in the recent history of the developed world and it differs widely across cultures. One survey of traditional societies (Whiting & Child, 1953) found large variations in the timing, severity and preferred methods of toilet-training practices, with an American sample of the time tending towards the harsh end of the spectrum. Training was not begun until almost 5 years in one African culture, but full bladder and bowel control was expected by 6 months of age among the Tanala of Madagascar. Training techniques ranged from the simple and indulgent ('you just tell the child what to do and he does it' among the Kwoma of New Guinea), through guided imitation, ridicule and beatings. The most striking continence curriculum was that of the Dahomeans of West Africa. Children who wet their sleeping mats were first beaten, but if this method failed a mixture of ash and water was poured over their heads and they were chased into the street by children singing 'Urine everywhere'. In one community, repeat offenders had a live frog attached to their waist, which reportedly frightened them into continence.

Historical variations in ways of dealing with incontinence are equally striking. Recommended cures for 'pyssying in the bedde' in the Middle Ages included consumption of ground hedgehog or powdered goat claw and having dried rooster combs sprinkled on the bed (Glicklich, 1951). Over the past century the West has seen pendulum swings between indulgence and severity, guided by a changing cast of child-rearing experts. At the beginning of the twentieth century a relaxed approach prevailed, based on the assumption that children would naturally achieve readiness for bladder and bowel control through a gradual process of maturation. This laissez-faire view gave way to stricter forms of training aimed at younger children (Luxem & Christophersen, 1994). Behaviourists such as James Watson understood continence as a set of habits that could be quickly taught through appropriate forms of conditioning. Under the influence of these ideas one American parenting magazine assured its readers in 1929 that training could be completed by 8 weeks of age.

By mid-century expert opinion began to swing back towards a permissive approach with the growing influence of psychoanalysis in the child guidance field and the views of psychologists such as Arnold Gesell, who emphasized the importance of the child's biological readiness for training. This more relaxed stance was promoted by the publication of Benjamin Spock's first baby- and child-care manual in 1946, which recommended that toilet training be child-centred and child-directed. Its subsequent editions shifted the recommended age for commencing toilet training later and later, enabled no doubt by the advent of washing machines and disposable nappies.

Toilet training plainly depends upon a combination of biological maturation and socialization – nature and nurture – and the relative importance of these factors has implications for the psychology of enuresis. Prolonged incontinence in children may reflect delayed physiological maturity or defective learning. Certain psychological attributes might also render some children vulnerable to developing enuresis, or might be residual signs or after-effects of it later in life. It is widely assumed that enuresis is psychologically meaningful and that children affected by it are emotionally troubled. This assumption reflects some of the early and mid-twentieth-century psychological accounts of enuresis, which viewed it as a sign of anxiety, unconscious resentment of the parents, or a desire to regress to infantile dependence. In boys it was sometimes taken to reveal a passive and effeminate personality, but in girls it was seen as demonstrating an unconscious striving for masculinity (Glicklich, 1951). In all of the theories, enuresis was interpreted as a symptom of something deeper, a leakage of some personal neurosis rather than a stand-alone behavioural problem.

In the case of nocturnal enuresis, or bed-wetting, there appears to be little truth to this view. The factors that contribute to it are primarily biological in nature and largely unrelated to temperament or psychological disturbance. Bed-wetting children often show signs of delayed physiological maturation, such as unstable sleep patterns (Martin et al., 1984), deficient release of a pituitary hormone (arginine vasopressin) that has an antidiuretic effect on kidney function and difficulty arousing from sleep when the bladder is full (Butler, 2001). Nocturnal enuresis also has a strong genetic component. Most studies find few differences if any between nocturnally enuretic and non-enuretic children in temperament or behavioural problems. A recent study found that nocturnal enuretic children aged 6 to 12 did not differ from unaffected children on any of the five major dimensions of personality or on the major dimensions of behavioural disturbance (Van Hoecke et al., 2006). Lasting effects of nocturnal enuresis are also minor, one Danish study finding that formerly enuretic young adults did not differ from their dry peers except in being somewhat more suspicious and more likely to feel that they did not belong in society (Strömgren & Thomsen, 1990).

The situation is less sanguine for two other groups of enuretics: those who are incontinent during the day and those who relapse after a period of established continence. These groups are known as diurnal and secondary enuretics, respectively. Secondary enuresis is a common regressive response to family difficulties such as parental separation and disharmony (Fergusson et al., 1990) as well as traumatic events. One-third of a sample of children in Bangladesh developed secondary enuresis after floods that devastated the country and left millions homeless in 1988 (Durkin et al., 1993). Diurnal enuretics also tend to have raised levels of psychological disturbance, although not always in response to specific life events. The same study that found no significant difference between nocturnal enuretics and unaffected children showed diurnal enuretics to be relatively neurotic, lacking in conscientiousness and self-confidence, and elevated on several measures of behaviour problems, including hyperactivity and deficiencies in sustained attention (Van Hoecke et al., 2006).

Enuresis evidently has a complicated relationship to psychological disturbance. Some forms appear to be almost entirely unrelated, caused instead by biological abnormalities and immaturities that have no direct link to emotional distress. Other forms are linked to neuroticism and deficient self-control, or express upset in response to stressful events. Whether or not incontinence is caused by unhappiness, it may nevertheless cause it. Children are usually embarrassed by their enuresis, keep it as a shameful secret, avoid social activities where it might be uncovered and suffer teasing if the secret leaks out. They know intuitively that incontinence is viewed as not just an unfortunate habit but a moral failing – a lack of the self-mastery that they *should* possess – and a humiliating return to infancy.

Bed-wetting and crime

Many myths surround bed-wetting and one of the most interesting is the idea that it might be related to criminal behaviour. Several psychiatrists have argued that bed-wetting is part of a triad of childhood behaviours, along with fire-setting and cruelty to animals, that predicts later delinquency and violence. Several early studies found support for the triad. Hellman and Blackman (1966) examined 84 adult male prisoners and showed that those who had been charged with aggressive crimes were almost three times as likely as those who had not to display all or part of the triad. Wax and Haddox (1974) found that 6 of a sample of 46 adolescent male offenders showed the full triad: these 6 all showed extreme violence and marked sexual deviation and were adjudged to be the most potentially dangerous in the youth authority. Evidence for the triad's prognostic value for women has also been obtained, with Felthous and Yudowitz (1977) showing that assaultive female prisoners had higher rates of enuresis, animal cruelty and fire-setting histories than their non-assaultive peers. Although the explanation for this apparent linkage between three dissimilar behaviours remains uncertain, one possibility is that all three reflect a congenital lack of self-restraint: a generalized form of incontinence.

Unfortunately for the triad, other studies have been less supportive. In the strongest of these, Heath and colleagues (1984) examined 204 consecutively admitted child psychiatry outpatients and recorded their rates of enuresis, fire-setting and animal cruelty. These researchers found no simple associations among the three behaviours: bed-wetters were no more likely to be fire-setters than non-bed-wetters, and animal cruelty was also unrelated to fire-setting. Interestingly, among children who were not cruel to animals, bed-wetters were especially likely to be fire-setters, as were animal sadists among those children who were not bed-wetters. One reading of these complex findings is that there is no triad, only two overlapping dyads: undercontrolled children who wet their beds and set fires and hostile children who abuse animals and set fires. In any event, the evidence for either dyad having a strong relationship to criminality and violence is weak indeed, and the consensus among forensic psychologists is that enuresis and the triad as a whole have no meaningful relationship with violent offending.

Urinary perversion

In paruresis the bladder is bashful and inhibited and in enuresis it is ashamed and poorly controlled. In other conditions the bladder is brazen or at least the focus of shameless fascination. Although sexual fetishes most often involve items of clothing or parts of the body, they occasionally include unwholesome interest in bodily products such as urine. This 'paraphilia', to use current psychiatric terminology, is generally referred to as urolagnia or undinism, the latter term derived by the British sexologist Havelock Ellis from the name for mythological water nymphs.

Few cases of undinism have been reported in the modern psychiatric literature, but Denson (1982) describes a 17-year-old boy who had an assortment of urine-related habits. He would eat 'yellow spots' in snow, drink from unflushed girls' toilets while working as a school janitor and had sampled a bucket of horse urine. His understanding of adult sexual relations was that they were completed by an act of mutual urination. His treating psychiatrist speculated that the boy's fetishistic interest in urine derived from this mistaken sexual idea, so that his erotic fantasies became linked to it. Contact with urine would then be accompanied by sexual excitement, thereby reinforcing his perverse interest.

Another case of undinism involved a man who grew up as one of the 20 children of a highly neurotic prostitute. At the age of 10 he first took great pleasure in urinating on a laundry basket of his mother's clean clothes, a pleasure he frequently repeated and later extended to urinating on clean white sheets, his wife's underwear and unsuspecting women in theatres and crowds. He also cultivated a variety of additional paraphilias, including exhibitionism, voyeurism and transvestism. His psychoanalyst interpreted his behaviour as an outlet for sadistic and ambivalent feelings towards his mother, whom he loved but saw as dirty. Taking on a life of its own, his undinism towards other women continued to symbolize his desire to degrade his mother and expressed his disappointment with her soiled state (London, 1950).

Undinism may be rare, but is rumoured to have kept notorious company. One of the many psychological accounts of Adolf Hitler's psychology – alongside a multitude of psychiatric diagnoses – proposes that he was partial to the perversion. According to this interpretation it was the horror of having to take part in the practice that led his niece, Geli Raubal, to shoot herself in his bedroom. It has also been used to explain the high incidence of suicide and suicide attempts among the women with whom Hitler is thought to have been intimate. The people who spread this story about Hitler's perversion, chiefly the embittered former Nazi leader Otto Strasser, had personal reasons to discredit him (Rosenbaum, 1998) and the evidence for the claim is as slender and impossible to validate as many psychobiographical interpretations. All the same, it makes for a lively tale.

The boy who ate yellow snow's fetish involved tasting urine and Hitler's was rumoured to involve watching it. Other undinists favour different sense modalities. The French psychiatrist Auguste Tardieu describes the case of 'renifleurs', or sniffers, who would loiter outside female public toilets or skulk at the back doors of theatres in the hope of catching the scent of women's urine. The early American psychoanalyst Abraham Brill, Freud's first English translator, wrote of one sniffer who adjusted successfully after treatment by turning his sense of smell into a vocation and becoming a florist (Brill, 1932).

Undinism relates specifically to urine but it is possible to connect it to a broader class of urethral forms of sexuality (Bass, 1994). For whatever reason, these forms were especially popular among famous sexologists. Havelock Ellis, the nineteenth century's best-known sexologist, appears to have been an undinist himself. Alfred Kinsey of Kinsey Report fame, the most notorious sexologist of the twentieth century, preferred the urethral insertion of a toothbrush, bristles and all (Jones, 1997).

Conclusions

Like the bowel, the bladder's functions attract strong and diverse emotional responses. Although urination draws less disgust than defecation, it is just as strongly associated with anxiety, fear, embarrassment and shame, and just as intimately linked to trauma and life stress. As we have seen, the bladder has its own phobia, its own form of hysterical conversion, its own inhibition failures, and its own perversions and fetishes. These disturbances have their roots in an assortment of genetic vulnerabilities, childhood experiences, abusive environments and bizarre ideas. At first blush urination might seem to be psychologically as sterile and inconsequential as the liquid itself, but a closer look shows otherwise.

4
On Flatulence

Charles Darwin's life was a vale of sorrows. His mother died when he was a boy, three of his own children perished at an early age, and his great discovery of the theory of evolution by natural selection was met with hostility by prominent members of society and many of his fellow scientists. Through most of his adult life he also suffered mightily from disabling anxiety, depression and physical symptoms that included heart palpitations, eczema, vomiting and flatulence. In his mid-fifties he described the latter thus: 'For 25 years extreme spasmodic daily & nightly flatulence... every passage of flatulence preceded by ringing of ears, treading on air & vision' (Desmond & Moore, 1991, p. 531).

Flatulence is universal. For some it is a minor annoyance or embarrassment, for others a source of amusement and for an unfortunate few it is a terrible burden. For Darwin, flatulence was the symptom of a deep malaise which combined fear, fatigue and black pessimism. According to one psychiatric biographer (Bowlby, 1990), it was the psychosomatic expression of an anxiety disorder linked historically to his mother's early death, exacerbated in the present by life stresses, and caused directly by a tendency to hyperventilate, the relevance of which will soon become clear.

More often than not flatulence has kept more cheerful company than Darwin's. It has been a staple of comedy since the ancient Greeks, reaching a peak in the ribald humour of the Middle Ages (Allen, 2007). Famous farts are documented in Chaucer's *Canterbury Tales* and in the *Arabian Nights*. Flatulence reaches heights of comic absurdity in the work of François Rabelais (1564/1965), who describes a fictitious volume in the library of St Victor on *The art of farting decently in public* and whose creation, the giant Pantagruel, unleashes one great fart whose 'foul air created more than fifty-three thousand tiny men, dwarves and creatures of weird shape'. This spirit of high-spirited vulgarity, often directed by the young and powerless against authority figures and the well-bred, survives to this day in a thousand jokes, children's books and popular culture references.

Sober scholarship on flatulence has been less abundant. With barely concealed sadness, Furne and Levitt (1996) remark that flatulence 'has been the province of lay conjecture and scatological humour rather than serious scientific investigation' (p. 1633). For more than 35 years Levitt and colleagues have tried to remedy this state of affairs with an energetic programme of physiological research on flatulence, coining the term 'flatology' to dignify their quest (Levitt, 1980). The term has failed to catch on, but before we can tackle the psychology of flatulence we must review some elementary flatology.

The physiology of flatulence

Flatulence is primarily composed of five gases: nitrogen, oxygen, hydrogen, methane and carbon dioxide. Of these, hydrogen, methane and carbon dioxide are produced by the fermentation of poorly absorbed carbohydrates in the gut by hundreds of species of microbe, known collectively as the 'colonic flora'. The mixing proportions of these gases vary widely between people and over time. Smaller quantities of sulphur-containing gases – primarily hydrogen sulphide, methanethiol and dimethyl sulphide – are responsible for the foul smell of flatulence, a finding confirmed by two brave judges who judged the odour intensity of farts collected via rectal tube from 16 healthy participants fed scientifically controlled quantities of pinto beans and lactulose (Suarez et al., 1998). The same three sulphurous gases account for the offensive odour of morning breath (Suarez et al., 2000), a finding first reported at the 4th international conference on breath odour.

Large-scale studies of flatus production have not been undertaken, but existing research suggests that on average people pass gas about 10 times per day and about 100 millilitres at a time (Furne & Levitt, 1996). Passing gas 20 times per day has been suggested as the threshold of abnormality (Levitt et al., 1998). Flatulence frequency changes appreciably in response to dietary alterations, but there is a good deal of consistency in people's levels of flatus production: some people reliably fart more than others.

At the quantitative extreme are some people whose flatulence is prodigious. Levitt and colleagues (Levitt et al., 1998) present the case of a computer programmer who complained of excessive flatus and painful abdominal gas. He also observed that his stools effervesced, like aspirins in a glass of water. The patient kept meticulous records of each passage of gas, with frequencies usually exceeding 50 times per day and reaching a peak of 129. Levels such as these may be exceptional, but complaints of flatulence are very common in the general population. One representative survey of the French public found that 61 per cent reported digestive symptoms that were unlikely to result from physical illness and almost half of these complained of flatulence (Frexinos et al., 1998). Elevated rates of flatulence have been reported in a variety of physical and psychological conditions, including irritable bowel syndrome, mental retardation and autism (Smith et al., 2009).

The psychoanalysis of flatulence

Our brief flatological survey provides a descriptive foundation for our investigation, but it tells us nothing about the psychological causes and dynamics of the phenomenon. Not surprisingly, it was the psychoanalysts who first took the psychology of flatulence seriously. Freud's biographer Ernest Jones (1918) speculated on the relationship between farting and musical ability, and his close associate Sandor Ferenczi (1950) addressed the reasons why patients might pass wind during psychoanalytic sessions. Generally, he argued, this act was not motivated by a desire to insult the analyst – although it was often done when the patient was being difficult and resistant – but rather as an attempt to claim the prerogative of adulthood. In effect, the patient is simply expressing in a rebellious and non-verbal manner the desire to be treated as a grown-up. Lorand (1931) discusses a young man whose flatulence, often performed for the amusement of his friends, represented a similar form of rebellious aggression that was linked to a penchant for 'dirty' language. Kubie (1937) confirmed the similarities between flatulence and swearing, pointing out the aggressive gaseous suddenness of both.

Other analysts report cases in which flatulence was a key clinical problem. Etchegoyen (2005) discusses the case of a man who presented for treatment suffering from flatulence and gastric discomfort, and had a tendency to burp and fart during sessions, at times with apparent pride. The analyst interpreted the man's gaseousness as an unconscious identification with a pregnant woman, although the patient had an unfortunate tendency to fall asleep following interpretations such as these. The analysis took a total of nine and a half years, not counting three years of prior treatment that ended with the death of the patient's previous analyst. Baker (1994) describes a more leisurely, 15-year analysis of a fetishistic cross-dresser for whom flatulence was the most intractable symptom. This treatment ended successfully upon the patient's rejection of his 'idealization of the anal universe that he inhabited'.

The most thorough psychoanalytic investigation of flatulence was conducted by Merrill (1951), who describes a series of patients that, he argued, reveal a particular character type. The patients, all men, were arrogant, boastful, impulsive and quick-tempered. They underachieved and had troubled relationships with women and with their fathers. They also tended to be drawn to foul language, dirty stories, sadistic and scape-goating wit, and exhibitionistic public displays. One patient was renowned in college for farting loudly (a 'stertorous roar') and for lighting his farts for the amusement of friends. (The flammability of intestinal gas has its serious side, with 20 reports of patients suffering explosions during surgery or colonoscopy, including nine colon perforations and one death [Ladas et al., 2007].)

Another of Merrill's patients mastered the art of swallowing air, enabling him to produce at will farts so loud that they once awakened fraternity brothers sleeping on a third-floor balcony. Another bragged about being able to play tunes with his anus. As a child he revelled in the masculine power flatulence gave him to shock women such as his nursemaid, whose nose he learned to assault when she bent to tie his shoe-laces. He refined this power in adulthood to the point that in bed he would break wind in his wife's face while he slept and would become more flatulent when her conversation bored him.

Merrill concluded that these men had failed to identify adequately with their fathers and as a result lacked self-control and the capacity for personal achievement. Their flatulence was a malodorous attempt to achieve adult masculinity.

Aerophagia

These psychoanalytic contributions speculate on a few of the possible meanings, dynamics and developmental origins of flatulence for particular individuals. However, they have little say on the more mundane issues of whether any ways of thinking or behaving contribute to it as a general rule. One of the more intriguing findings about flatulence is that behaviour at the other end of the digestive system makes a major contribution to the quantity of intestinal gas. Any emotional states and psychological conditions that influence this behaviour may thereby promote flatulence. Although people tend to assume that flatus is exclusively brewed in the gut, it appears that ingested air is often a major source.

The truth of this statement was brought home forcefully in the case of Levitt and colleagues' (1998) farting prodigy. Under the sway of the intestinal theory of flatulence he had tried without success a large number of treatments that aimed to reduce, supplement or fertilize the colonic flora, including medications, herbal supplements, charcoal and assorted diets. Levitt and colleagues took careful and repeated measurements of the composition of his rectal gas and found concentrations of nitrogen that were close to atmospheric levels. As nitrogen is not a product of colonic fermentation they concluded that the man's flatulence largely resulted from air swallowing, or 'aerophagia'.

Aerophagia is a troublesome symptom that is often accompanied by frequent belching, abdominal pain and distension, and subjective bloating. It has been linked to a wide variety of psychological conditions. It is commonly observed among people with intellectual disability and developmental delays (Van der Kolk, 1999), and one case has been reported in which aerophagic behaviour was so severe that it resulted in perforation of a boy's colon, with serious medical complications (Basaran et al., 2007). Case reports have linked the onset of serious aerophagia to depression (Appleby & Rosenberg, 2006; D'Mello, 1983). Aerophagic patients also tend to be highly anxious and have higher levels of anxiety than patients suffering from other gastrointestinal conditions (Chitkara et al., 2005). Air-swallowing has also been observed in a case of obsessive-compulsive disorder (Zella et al., 1998): a 9-year-old girl who belched compulsively in response to obsessive fears that she might vomit, and who would stimulate her belches by gulping carbonated drinks. Flatulence was a significant side effect. Aerophagia can also be a consequence of involuntary vocal tics in Tourette's syndrome (Frye & Hait, 2006; Weil et al., 2008).

The swallowing of air also occurs outside the context of psychological disturbance. All of us ingest quantities of air when we eat, drink and swallow saliva. For example, it has been estimated that for every litre of liquid consumed, 1.7 litres of air are ingested. Rapid eaters and infants who suck thumbs or toes may be especially prone to this kind of incidental aerophagia. Large surveys have shown that air-swallowing is one of the most common gastrointestinal symptoms that people report (Drossman, 1993) and it appears to be responsive to people's emotional state. Spontaneous rates of air-swallowing increase when people are anxious or under cognitive stress (Fonagy, 1986), and one study found a threefold increase in swallowing when people were placed in unpleasantly arousing situations (Cuevas et al., 1995). Much of the ingested air may be exhaled as belches, but the remainder runs the risk of contributing to flatulence. The source of Charles Darwin's flatulence may have been in his anxious hyperventilation.

Successful treatment of aerophagia with a variety of psychotropic medications has been reported, with anti-anxiety and antidepressant drugs most often used. Psychological treatments have also been effective, including hypnosis and psychotherapy. Direct forms of behaviour modification may also be effective. Patients can be made aware of their air-swallowing, which may have been unconscious, with the aid of a throat microphone, and they can be taught methods to control it (Calloway et al., 1983). These include breathing exercises (Cigrang et al., 2006), muscle relaxation, self-administration of electric shocks upon belching, positive reinforcement for non-aerophagic behaviour and the performance of substitute behaviours that are incompatible with swallowing (e.g., covering the mouth with the hand [Garcia et al., 2001] or gently biting the forefinger in the case of one successfully treated 4-year-old boy [Flaisher, 1994]). Although all of these treatments target the mouth, they would be expected to have positive effects at the other end of the alimentary tube.

On the subject of psychological treatments, it should be noted that those targeting irritable bowel syndrome also commonly show effectiveness in reducing flatulence. Anti-flatulent effects have been demonstrated by a variety of treatments involving group cognitive therapy (Blanchard et al., 2007), behaviour therapy (Schwarz et al., 1990), hypnosis (Galovski & Blanchard, 1998) and relaxation-based meditation (Keefer & Blanchard, 2001). In sum, flatulence is not simply the physical product of a troubled biology, but has a psychological component that can be treated by psychological means.

Flatulence and emotion

Flatulence and depression

Links between flatulence and depression have long been suggested. The Greek physician Aretaeus of Cappadocia, who practised in the first century AD, associated melancholy with flatulence in a very literal fashion, proposing that excesses of black bile, from which melancholia gets its name, directly cause depression: 'If it [black bile] be determined upwards to the stomach and diaphragm, it forms melancholy; for it produces flatulence and eructations of a fetid and fishy nature, and it sends rumbling wind downwards, and disturbs the understanding.' In joining flatulence and belching (eructation) Aretaeus anticipated the association between flatulence and aerophagia that was scientifically established about two millennia later. His clinical observation of the adverse effects of flatulence on mental focus backs up the dietary restrictions of the Pythagoreans, who according to Cicero were forbidden to eat beans 'for that food induces flatulence and induces a condition at war with a soul in search of truth' (Bailey, 1961).

Robert Burton, the British scholar who wrote *The anatomy of melancholy* in the early seventeenth century, also drew attention to a correlation between melancholia and wind. Referring to a hypochondriacal form of depression, he wrote: 'In this kind of Melancholy one of the most offensive symptoms is wind, which, as in other species, so in this, hath great need to be corrected and expelled' (Burton, 1621/1850, p. 418). One radical treatment that he described for those troubled by 'flatuous melancholy' was to 'put a pair of bellows' end into a Clyster [enema] pipe, and applying it into the fundament, open the bowels, so draw forth the wind; nature abhors a vacuum' (p. 419). Writing a century later, George Cheyne (1733/1976), a Scottish physician who treated such notables as David Hume, Samuel Johnson and Alexander Pope, proposed in *The English malady* that depression-like diseases were associated with flatulence and a sense of oppression and anxiety. He describes a distemper of 'vapours' in which 'the symptoms... besides lowness of spirits, are wind, belching, yawning, heart-burning, croaking of the bowels, (like the noise of frogs), a pain in the pit of the stomach' and so on (p. 136).

There is a lack of systematic research on the association between flatulence and depression in more recent times. Haug and colleagues (2002, 2004) found a relationship between levels of depression and gastrointestinal symptoms including constipation and diarrhoea in the general population, but did not examine flatulence itself. Martens et al. (2010) found high rates of depressive and anxiety symptoms in patients presenting with a diverse assortment of gastrointestinal problems with a presumed psychological basis. As we saw earlier, depression has been linked to aerophagia (Appleby & Rosenberg, 2006; D'Mello, 1983) and thereby to the likelihood of significant flatulence. However, the existence of a specific connection between depression and flatulence remains uncertain.

Flatulence and fear

Flatulence appears to be linked to diffuse anxiety and other forms of neurotic misery, but it is also associated with highly focused fears. Several writers have reported cases of individuals suffering from profound fears of flatulence, which sometimes reached delusional intensity. These fears take interestingly different forms. Ladouceur et al. (1993) and Lyketsos (1992) present cases of men whose obsessive fears centred on the social offence that public flatulence would cause and led to anxiety attacks and social withdrawal. The former case was resolved through behaviour therapy whereas the second responded to antidepressant medication. Fears of flatulence with a less directly social focus were discussed by Kubota (1987), who used a form of hypnotic treatment to overcome fears of flatulence in an adolescent Japanese girl. Her dread was conceptualized as 'automysophobia', the pathological fear of being dirty. Unlike the previous cases, this patient saw flatulence more as a way of soiling herself than as causing affront to others. Similarly, the case of a young man with obsessive concerns about flatulence, reported by Fishbain and Goldberg (1991) and successfully treated with antidepressants, revolves around a fear of loss of personal control more than loss of social face.

Beary and Cobb (1981) describe three cases that are different again, each patient having a delusional conviction that they emitted an 'alimentary stench' (flatulence or bad breath). Cases of this sort are sometimes traceable to specific smell-related events, such as being teased after breaking wind (Begum & McKenna, 2011). After the delusions first develop they are frequently reinforced by the patient's continual misreading of other people's behaviour, for example seeing their innocent gifts of perfume as not-so-subtle hints, or taking their sniffing or coughing – and even the barking of nearby dogs – as evidence of one's foul odour. Patients often compensate for their imagined stench by avoiding social situations, compulsively checking their smell and overusing deodorants and soaps. Beary and Cobb treated their patients with moderate success by exposing them to situations they avoided and preventing them from engaging in their habitual compensatory behaviour.

One intriguing but rarely used way of treating obsessive thoughts about flatulence involves encouraging farting rather than preventing it. Milan and Kolko (1982), using this 'paradoxical intention' method, instructed a female patient to pass wind as soon as the urge to do so arose, and the reduction in ruminative thoughts about flatulence that resulted persisted for at least one year.

Flatulence and disgust

Depression and fear play their roles in the psychology of flatulence, but the emotion of disgust is perhaps the most intimately related to it. Disgust is a basic emotion evolved in response to stimuli that threaten contamination and disease, such as excrement and decaying food and bodies. It is easily evoked by the chemical senses of odour and taste, and its typical facial expression involves wrinkling the nose to close off the nostrils. Psychologists have recently begun to harness the power of smell to induce disgust in their experiments. The preferred tool for this purpose is fart spray, which is commercially available from novelty stores and more commonly purchased by 13-year-old boys than older scientists.

In one of the first scientific uses of flatulent technology, Schnall and colleagues (2008) exposed their participants to different intensities of spray: unlucky participants were randomly assigned to a 'strong stink' condition and luckier participants to 'mild stink' and non-stink 'control' conditions. The former reported higher levels of disgust than the latter. Participants then rated how objectionable a variety of morally questionable acts would be, such as marriage or consensual sex between first cousins. Participants who were exposed to the fart spray expressed stronger moral condemnation for several of the acts, just as people have been shown to become more morally judgemental when disgust is induced by hypnosis (Wheatley & Haidt, 2005). It seems that when a strong feeling of distaste is evoked, even by a purely sensory experience, a variety of social violations come to be seen as more distasteful or disgusting as well. This creates a special problem for anyone who farts in public: the evidence of their offence is likely to magnify the perceived offensiveness of the act in the eyes (or nose) of a witness.

It is not only the smell of flatulence that can have psychological effects. Recent work (Davey et al., 2006; Mayer et al., 2009) has experimentally induced disgust with a mixture of fart, vomit and burp noises, combined with images of a filthy toilet. These researchers found that disgust created a negative bias in people's judgement of ambiguous situations, leading them to interpret these situations as more threatening than do people who are placed in neutral or happy moods.

One idle question we might ask is whether people find the scent of their own flatulence less offensive than others'. Sadly no rigorous studies have been conducted. The closest evidence comes from a study of mothers' judgements of the offensiveness of faeces-soiled nappies (Case et al., 2006). Mothers asked to smell concealed samples of their own baby's nappies judged them less disgusting than those of another baby, even when the labels of the respective samples were deceptively switched. Similar findings have been obtained in studies of perceptions of armpit odours, where people prefer their own scent and those of close relations to those of strangers (Levine & McBurney, 1986). This may be a simple case of habituation: familiarity breeds liking, or at least tolerance, rather than contempt. However, it may also be functional. If parents have strong disgust reactions to their own infants they may be unable to care for them with sufficient thoroughness. No similar function can be easily imagined for a preference for one's own flatulence, but there is now at least some indirect evidence that we may tend to underestimate its offensiveness relative to the emanations of others.

Defensive flatulence

The disgusting quality of flatulence generally motivates people to inhibit it in public places and to condemn those who fail to do so. It is this fear of embarrassment and blame that minimizes the passage of gas when other people are present. But might there be cases where people harness the disgusting power of farts to keep people at a distance? Just as skunks use foul odours to defend and protect themselves, might people do the same?

There is only one clinical report of apparently deliberate skunk-like behaviour in a human. Mara Sidoli (1996), a Jungian psychoanalyst, presents the case of a young boy who, she argued, used flatulence to form a 'defensive olfactory container' or envelope to protect himself from fears of disintegration. Peter had been born to an alcohol-abusing teenage mother and fostered out at an early age. He had severe feeding problems as an infant, was neglected and abused as a child, and underwent numerous surgeries for a variety of ailments. His main symptoms upon entering therapy at age 7 included manic hyperactivity, confused speech, conversations with imaginary beings and loud farts and (oral) farting noises. Sidoli inferred that Peter had profound abandonment fears and fantasies of persecution, the latter often represented in his play as attacks by space aliens. His farting intensified during times of anxiety and anger, a symptom that Sidoli interpreted as an attempt to emit a 'protective cloud of familiarity', creating an invisible barrier preventing harm as well as communication with the world outside.

A turning point in Peter's analysis occurred when Sidoli, presumably departing from normal psychoanalytic practice, began to make loud farting noises back at him. Peter's initial response was surprise followed by intense anger, during which he called Sidoli crazy, but he soon began laughing himself. Sidoli argues that by showing Peter how crazy and annoying his behaviour seemed to others and interpreting to him that by acting in this way he had been trying to drive people away by acting crazy, she helped to loosen his defences.

Sure enough, his flatulence began to subside and his aggressiveness began to give way to greater warmth and engagement with others: 'instead of enveloping me with farts, he was able to show me his pain' (p. 178).

Enjoyment of flatulence

Up to this point I have emphasized links between flatulence, psychopathology and negative emotions. However, farting can also be a source of amusement. Flatulence is the focus of countless jokes and humorous stories. The act itself is often greeted with laughter and even elaborated into ribald contests and pyrotechnic displays, especially by pre-adolescent boys (and those developmentally arrested at that stage; Merrill, 1951). Psychologists have paid little systematic attention to the ludic aspects of flatulence, but Lippman (1980) has made a preliminary study. He presented a sample of college students with a description of a hypothetical fart that varied on four dimensions – relationship between the farter and witnesses (acquaintances or strangers), intention (deliberate or accidental), sound (loud or nearly silent) and odour (very rank or almost odourless) – and had them judge how humorous it would be. Farts were adjudged more humorous when deliberately, loudly, but odourlessly committed in the presence of acquaintances.

Lippman also asked participants to judge the politeness, maliciousness and obnoxiousness of flatulence under the 16 possible combinations of the four factors. Farts were judged most polite when accidental, silent, odourless and among acquaintances, and most malicious and obnoxious under the opposite combination: deliberate, loud, rank and in the presence of strangers. Consistent with this pattern, in a second section of the study participants said they would be most likely to try to suppress an imminent passage of gas if it was likely to be loud, smelly and amid strangers, as well as when they could probably be identified as its source. Interestingly, then, farts are most humorous when they are halfway between politeness and obnoxiousness: odourless and in the presence of acquaintances, like polite breakings of wind, but also loud and deliberate, like malicious ones. They are potentially embarrassing but not outright shameful, the potential for humour being one of the elements that distinguishes awkward embarrassment from toxic shame (Tangney et al.,

1996). In short, the humorousness of flatulence may derive from a controlled violation of social norms of propriety. As Merrill (1951) puts it: 'Wit itself, Freud pointed out, is a sudden overwhelming of the superego. This . . . is the very essence of flatulence' (p. 559).

Flatulence and gender

Our final topic is the possibility of sex differences related to flatulence. There appear to be some differences in production. Furne and Levitt (1996) found no difference between male and female participants in the frequency of flatulence, but other researchers (Suarez et al., 1998) discovered that women's flatulence was on average lesser in volume but greater in olfactory offensiveness than men's. The latter effect also appears to hold for morning breath (Snel et al., 2011), with women showing higher concentrations of the sulphur compounds that contribute to unpleasant odour.

Other sex differences may involve discrepancies in the manner in which flatulence is expressed, inhibited and disapproved. There is little scientific work on this subject and even apparent experts in human psychology seem to lack confident knowledge of it. Like an anthropologist observing the strange behaviour of an exotic tribe, one male psychiatrist remarked that 'it would seem that women when not alone customarily pass gas silently' (Merrill, 1951, p. 558). There is some empirical basis for his claim that women are more reticent when it comes to flatulence. Weinberg and Williams (2005) found that heterosexual men were three times as likely as heterosexual women to report often engaging in intentional flatulence and twice as likely to find faecal noises funny. Heterosexual women were more likely than heterosexual men to think overhearers would find faecal sounds disgusting, and much more likely to think that being overheard making these sounds would affect their relationship with the overhearer. These differences appear to be about gender, gender-related social roles and sexuality rather than biological sex itself. For example, gay men were less likely to report intentionally passing gas than heterosexual women, and lesbians were more likely. Differences between the sexes in flatulence-related attitudes and practices seem to be a matter of stereotypical masculinity and femininity.

Weinberg and Williams (2005) speculate at length on the gendered meanings of 'fecal habits' and flatulence. They argue that women have a heightened concern for purity and cleanliness, in part due to the idealization of their bodies and stigmatization of its products. As a result they avoid the subject of elimination and are more preoccupied with deodorization and keeping their excretion hidden and private. Indeed, within their sample heterosexual women were substantially more bothered than men by using public restrooms and more likely to think that having their faecal noises overheard would imply that they were not meeting a gender ideal.

Women may feel more disgust and shame about flatulence and other faecal phenomena than men and seek to suppress and distance themselves from them more, but this is not the whole story of the gender difference. Men at times seem to actively flout social norms governing faecal matters and doing so seems to be a way of performing their masculinity. Weinberg and Williams (2005) suggest that among men 'bodily grossness may be valued for its opposition to the manners that femininity is thought to imply' (p. 317). One of their heterosexual male participants expressed this colourfully when asked how others might feel if they smelled his flatulence: 'Guys would say it's raunchy and then say "Nice one," because if it's strong it's more manly. You know, because women would not try to clear a room with a fart' (p. 328). Ostentatious farting and burping is a way to assert male privilege and to breach codes of conduct that are seen as overly restrictive, middle-class, womanly and mature. In psychoanalytic language Merrill (1951) made the same point, proposing that his pathological farters were engaged in an aggressive form of 'counterphobic exhibitionism', a public display of masculine resistance to social prohibitions. Lippman (1980) went so far as to refer to farts as 'male weapons'.

The gendered nature of attitudes to flatulence is played out in humour. Women have traditionally found flatulence-related humour less amusing than men. Although Lippman (1980) found no overall difference between male and female college students in the rated humorousness of farts, he did find that women were less amused by their more disgusting aspects, seeing less humour in faecal odours. This tendency is consistent with a tendency for women to be less taken by and less likely to engage in humour that focuses on the body and its products (Kotthoff, 2006). It is equally consistent with men's tendency to be more disposed to enjoy aggressive humour, such as sarcasm, teasing and disparagement (Martin et al., 2003). It is noteworthy that vocal farting noises – variously known as raspberries or Bronx cheers – are at least superficially humorous ways of disparaging others, and also that men tend to see farts as more malicious than do women (Lippman, 1980). The disposition to enjoy more aggressive forms of humour is associated not just with stereotypically masculine traits of cynicism, hostility and competitiveness, but also with the absence of stereotypically feminine traits of understanding, warmth and kindness, just as Weinberg and Williams (2005) proposed that men's deliberate bodily grossness partly reflects a repudiation of things feminine.

Conclusions

The subject of flatulence might seem frivolous and merely titillating. However, we have seen that it has a serious side and reveals numerous psychological complexities. It is intimately connected to many forms of psychopathology, ranging from disorders of mood and anxiety to delusional psychotic conditions, severe developmental problems, tic disorders and disorders of personality. It has a remarkable capacity to evoke the full spectrum of human emotions, from embarrassment and shame, disgust and contempt, fear and sadness, to happiness and laughter. It illuminates some of the baffling subtleties of the psychology of gender. Who would have thought that the links between wind and mind would be so intriguing?

5
The Anal Character

Psychoanalysis is the most breathtakingly ambitious psychological theory. It aspires to account for human cognition, emotion, motivation and culture, as well as explaining the causes of mental illness and the methods of treating it. As a theory of personality it offers elaborate models of the mind's levels of consciousness, the conflicting agencies that make it up and the tortuous stages through which personality develops. Although it is chiefly a theory of the dynamics of personality – the hidden processes that underlie human behaviour – it also contains a less well-known account of personality description. Freud and his followers proposed a small number of character types, each named after a body part. The most interesting is the anal character.

Freud's theory of character is intimately connected to his model of human development. On Freud's account, the child progresses through a series of stages that are psychosexual in nature, each one linked to a zone of bodily pleasure and a corresponding mode of relating to the world. In the oral stage the infant literally derives nourishment as well as sensual enjoyment from sucking, and it is also metaphorically concerned with ingesting and incorporating new experiences. In the anal stage the toddler derives pleasure from exercising its sphincters and its growing ability to hold on and let go, and is also preoccupied more broadly with self-control and exerting its will. In the phallic stage, the pre-school child's sexuality shifts focus to its genitals and the psychosexual development of boys and girls starts to diverge.

According to psychoanalytic theory, this progression from organ to organ is rarely straightforward and difficulties encountered while navigating a stage will leave their mark on the future adult. Fixations in particular stages leave the person vulnerable to distinctive forms of mental illness, distinctive ways of perceiving others and signature methods of dealing with external threats and internal impulses: in short, they leave an impression on the person's character. Fixations in the anal stage, caused by harsh toilet training in particular or more generally by parental thwarting of the child's growing autonomy, may lead the child to develop an anal character.

Freud first identified the anal character in 1908. In a short paper entitled 'Character and anal erotism', he noted a cluster of three traits which has come to be known as the anal triad: orderliness, obstinacy and parsimony. Orderliness referred to conscientiousness, reliability and a concern with cleanliness; obstinacy involved stubbornness, wilfulness and irascibility; and parsimony amounted to a tight and miserly way with money, which, Freud, argued, is often symbolically equated with faeces, especially when it takes the form of gold.

Freud observed that these traits co-occur not only with one another, but also with a pattern of concern with defecation. He observed that people with the traits tended to recall having derived pleasure as infants from emptying their bowels and also from 'holding back'. These signs of intensified 'erotogenic significance' of the anus do not persist into adulthood and Freud inferred that anal character traits form as sublimations of the child's earlier wishes or as reaction-formations against them. That is, the obsessive cleanliness and scrupulous morality of anal characters are reactions against their unseemly childhood interest in filth and their wilfulness and tightness with money are socially acceptable expressions of their earlier struggles over toilet training and faecal retention.

Freud merely sketched the anal character and it was left to two psychoanalytic pioneers, Ernest Jones (1918/1950) and Karl Abraham (1923), to complete the portrait. Were the term not already reserved, we might be tempted to name these three pioneers the 'anal triad'. Jones seconded Freud's view that this character type originated in the infant's interest in defecation, arguing that it begins life with a thoroughly positive attitude towards its faeces and that the repression of these coprophilic interests and pleasures produces anal traits.

Jones and Abraham both catalogued the manifestations of these three traits. Orderliness is revealed in perfectionism, pedantry, an obsession with formalities, a passion for classifying and organizing, an exaggerated tendency for disgust and a concern with contamination, and a strong but inflexible sense of duty, thoroughness and efficiency. Obstinacy is demonstrated by a strong concern with maintaining personal control, with a firm sense of independence and personal uniqueness, and with a resentful sensitivity to interference and encroachment by others. Parsimony takes the form of meanness with money, being reluctant to borrow or lend, avarice, hoarding worthless objects and collecting. Jones opined that 'all collectors are anal-erotics' (p. 430) and tend to amass such 'copro-symbols' as coins and books. According to Otto Fenichel (1945) parsimony could also be temporal, in the form of attitudes towards punctuality and a concern with 'wasting' time.

In addition to their careful dissection of anal personality traits, Jones and Abraham proposed several more specific habits and tendencies associated with this character type. Jones observed that anal characters are often 'notorious bores' who are hard to get along with at work and are unable to delegate. They often procrastinate on tasks but then brook no interruption when they start to carry them out. They have fine handwriting. They take everything too seriously and 'their life is a never-ending struggle to get things right' (p. 422). Abraham agreed on the subject of the joylessness of anal characters, suggesting that 'they make up the main army of malcontents' (p. 407) and are often afflicted with 'Sunday neurosis', an unhappiness about having to interrupt their work and enjoy leisure.

Some of the features said to be associated with the anal character seem a little more far-fetched. Jones supposed that anal characters are intensely curious about the reverse side of things, such as what is on the other side of a hill; they frequently mistake left and right; they are fascinated with underground passages and tunnels; they are preoccupied with finding the centre of things; and they may have a tendency not to change underclothing 'more than is absolutely necessary' (p. 429). Abraham added that anal characters tended to take pleasure in keeping time-sheets and in 'all kinds of statistics' (p. 406). Some of them, he thought, display a chronic widening of the nostrils due to frequent raising of their upper lips, as if they were constantly sniffing something. Others display their parsimony through an extremely sparing use of toilet paper.

The picture of the anal character presented by Freud, Jones and Abraham is decidedly ambivalent. They pull no punches on the type's limitations – it makes the person 'exceedingly unfitted for social relations' (Jones, 1918/1950, p. 437) – and suggest that it puts people at risk of developing paranoia and obsessional neurosis, now known as obsessive-compulsive disorder. On the other hand, the three analysts also recognize the type's strengths. At their best, anal characters are determined, persistent in the face of obstacles, independent-minded, reliable, organized, efficient and thorough. These are decidedly modern virtues: individualist, work-obsessed, productive and economical.

Post-Freudian developments

Later psychoanalytic writers took the anal character in new directions, expanding its meaning, placing primary emphasis on different facets and substituting less anatomical names. Wilhelm Reich (1933/1949), who later found notoriety for discovering 'orgone', a sexual life energy that he believed could cure cancer and coax rain from clouds, described a 'compulsive' character type in which people were robot-like 'living machines'. David Shapiro (1965) identified a related type of character, the obsessive-compulsive, whose key features were rigidity, a rule-bound way of living, intellectuality and an aquiline focus on detail. People with this 'neurotic style' have a way of thinking and perceiving that amounts to failing to see the forest for the trees.

Erich Fromm (1947), whose neo-Freudianism emphasized the social and political dimensions of psychoanalysis, developed his own set of six character types. One of these, the 'hoarding orientation', described those who see other people and things as possessions to be collected and saved rather than shared. Fromm characterized this type with such unmistakably anal traits as 'orderly', 'methodical', 'stingy', 'stubborn' and 'pedantic'.

Erik Erikson (1963) saw the origins of these traits in the toddler's maturing control of its body's musculature and in the struggles between its will and the authoritative demands of its parents. These struggles may be dramatized in the process of toilet training but cannot be reduced to this anal arena. For Erikson, the anal character is simply one form of unsatisfactory passage through a stage of development in which the child strives for autonomy but risks being overcome by shame, riddled with doubt and apt to develop an overly rigid conscience as a way of coping. The extent to which the child can exercise its autonomy without being shamed and made to question itself ultimately boils down to how its parents wield their control.

Erikson did not hesitate to hold societal forces responsible for children's difficulties in this regard: it is 'the spread of middle-class mores', 'the ideal image of the mechanized body' and the belief that rigorous child training is 'absolutely necessary for the development of orderliness and punctuality' (p. 81) that produce anal traits. Norman Brown (1968) went further and viewed the anal character as one manifestation of the spirit of capitalism. For writers such as these the anal character became less a clinical description of disturbed individuals than a political critique of a disturbed society.

Applying the anal character

Psychoanalysts have put the concept of the anal character to use extensively in clinical case studies, analyses of cultural phenomena and psychobiographies. One example of the first is the case of an elderly paranoid woman described by Berkeley-Hill (1921), whose personality was described as obstinate, neat and orderly, and who had a habit of collecting shiny pebbles and other items that she referred to as 'jewels' in a colon-shaped bag, complete with a puckered, rectal opening. Anal themes in culture have been examined by psychoanalytic folklorists such as Alan Dundes (1978), who found evidence of them in American football ('protecting the endzone' and the like) and in the supposed preoccupation of German culture with order and cleanliness, as well as its supposed fondness for symbolically faecal foods (e.g., sausage) and flatulent music (i.e., wind and brass) (Dundes, 1984). (Recent research casts some doubt on the last claim, finding that players of wind and brass instruments are in fact less conscientious than string players [Langendorfer, 2008].) Even beloved fairy tales, such as 'The three bears', have yielded to anal interpretations (Elms, 1977). Goldilocks, a disorderly girl whose hair colour, according to Freud, Jones and others, commonly symbolizes faeces, encounters several fastidious woodland creatures who are intensely bothered by her slight disruptions to their porridge and beds. To make matters worse, her posterior wreaks havoc on their chairs.

One of the most thorough applications of the concept of the anal character is in a psychoanalytically informed biography of Richard Nixon, the 37th President of the USA, who resigned in disgrace in 1974 following the Watergate affair. Vamik Volkan and colleagues (1997) diagnosed a number of anal elements in Nixon's psychological make-up. According to their analysis, he was an inveterate collector of intelligence about political opponents and family members, and of a frequently recited list of unprecedented achievements. The White House tapes revealed him as prone to discharge dirty words in an obsessive fashion. His preoccupation with leaks of information from his office was interpreted as a fear of loss of control and symbolically equated with faecal incontinence. Colleagues described his personality as compulsive and his psychobiographers characterize him as someone who habitually used the anal defence of intellectualization to deal with the messiness of human emotion.

Research on the anal character

As we have seen, the anal character is a long-established concept that has played a significant role in psychoanalytic theory and practice. Analysts have assembled a diverse set of traits into an elaborate description of this personality type. People with anal characters are said to be orderly, neat, self-disciplined, preoccupied with cleanliness and troubled by dirt and disorder. They are said to be stubborn, preoccupied with control, rigid and fiercely protective of their personal autonomy. They are stingy, punctual and prone to hoard and collect. They are pathologically detail-focused, emotionally constricted, moralistic, self-righteous, intolerant and defend themselves from perceived threats by intellectualizing.

This portrait of the anal character is richly detailed. It is also entirely impressionistic, a product of clinical observation and theory rather than empirical research. If the anal character is to have scientific legitimacy it must be shown to be real. That task was taken up by a number of psychoanalytically informed researchers in the middle of the twentieth century. It was no simple task, because it involves several distinct research questions. First and most basically, do the proposed features of the anal character really cohere as Freud and others have argued? That is, at a purely descriptive level, do so-called anal traits co-vary with one another in such a way that they form a unified personality type? If the traits do not in fact co-occur – if the triad does not triangulate – then it makes little sense to refer to them as a distinct kind of character.

A second research question is also descriptive, but goes a little deeper. Freud and his followers did not merely propose that an anal character type existed, but theorized that it was related to defecation. It is important to ask whether there is, in fact, anything anal about the anal character. Even if the description of the anal character is a masterfully accurate psychological portrait, it is entirely possible that it has no special relationship with attitudes or impulses related to defecation. For Freud, of course, this connection between the character type and its anatomical region was fundamental: anal characters had distinctive excretory and coprophilic habits as children and these left an unconscious residue that found expression in their adult personalities.

A third research question is explanatory rather than descriptive. Freud and his acolytes maintained that anal characters were produced, at least in part, through struggles over toilet training. By their account, childhood battles over the socialization of excretion – submitting to parental authority versus wilfully defying it – are at the root of adult obstinacy. Similarly, the adult's orderliness and cleanliness and the disgust and shame that underlie them, originate in repression of the child's coprophilia brought about by strict toilet training. To test the psychoanalytic account of the anal character, it is necessary to investigate whether the harshness of toilet training in childhood is, in fact, associated with the anal traits in adulthood.

Do anal traits cohere?

A number of empirical research studies have investigated whether anal traits correlate with one another as Freud's description of the anal character would suggest. The evidence on this score is largely supportive. An early study by Sears (1936) found that questionnaire measures of anal triad traits were correlated with one another among adults. Later work by Barnes (1952) was equally encouraging, indicating that the traits such as orderliness, reliability, meticulousness, cleanliness and obedience to laws go together. Since that time, several researchers have been successful in developing tests of anal personality traits and providing evidence that these traits systematically co-occur. Grygier (1961) produced a questionnaire measure of six anal traits including hoarding, attention to detail, rigidity, submissiveness to authority, sadism and insularity, and researchers who have used it have established that most of these scales correlate with one another. Lazare and colleagues (1966) developed a test of 'obsessive' personality that assessed a constellation of anal traits, including orderliness, parsimony, obstinacy, rigidity, perseverance and emotional constriction. Kline (1969) developed perhaps the best-known scale of this type, using it to show, among other things, that science students score higher than arts students.

Other researchers have established correlations between specific anal traits in a more piecemeal fashion. Pettit (1969) showed an association between a measure of anal traits and measures of lack of spontaneity and an anal approach to time, such as endorsing the value of punctuality and sentiments such as 'Time is money'. Hetherington and Brackbill (1963) found some degree of association between measures of obstinacy and orderliness, but not miserliness, among 5-year-old girls, using an inventive assortment of tasks. Obstinacy was assessed by the child's persistence on tedious and ritualistic tasks, orderliness by ratings of the neatness of the child's kindergarten locker and the meticulousness of her finger-painting, and miserliness by the child's tendency to hoard gravel in a shoe-box.

The evidence in support of our first research question, the coherence of anal traits, is therefore quite strong. There is something unified and real about the character type that Freud first described and that Abraham, Jones and later psychoanalysts embroidered.

Are anal traits really 'anal'?

Even if it is true that anal traits form a tight and coherent cluster, however, it is not necessarily true that this cluster is 'anal' in any meaningful sense. For this to be true, people who are unusually orderly, obstinate and parsimonious would have to have some usual relationship to faeces in particular or perhaps, if we can be a little lenient and metaphorical, with filth in general. Several studies have pointed to a link of this sort. Templer and colleagues (1984) developed a measure of 'body elimination attitude' to assess disgust with bodily wastes and examined whether it was associated with measures of anal traits. The new measure – which contained items inquiring about such matters as being bothered by faecal odours, animal droppings, dirty ears and nasal discharge – was indeed elevated among people scoring high on an obsessiveness scale, as well as among women, the less educated and people without children. A similar association was found by Juni (1984), who showed that compulsive people professed relatively high levels of disgust, both towards those who violate 'anal' expectations for hygiene (e.g., 'people who don't bathe or shower') and towards oral offenders (e.g., 'people who slurp their soup').

The most memorable study of this type was conducted by Rosenwald and colleagues (1966), who asked whether people with conflicts around anal issues would have difficulty coping with situations that evoke anal anxieties. Participants in their study had to perform a hand–eye coordination task – identifying by touch submerged metal objects from a few visually presented alternatives – while their arms were plunged elbow-deep into two different media. They first completed the task with objects submerged in water and then repeated the task with different objects submerged in a thick and malodorous mixture of used crankcase oil and flour, described by the researchers as a 'fecal-like stimulus'. The researchers supposed that people with poorly resolved anal conflicts would not cope well with this disgusting challenge and would as a result perform more poorly on it than when they did the same task in water. Sure enough, people whose performance declined in the faecal version of the task tended to be indecisive and performed poorly on a task requiring mental flexibility. By implication, their 'anal' personalities played a role in their responses to faecal phenomena.

Links between anal traits and these phenomena have also been obtained in a study that used a controversial personality test known as the Blacky Pictures, in which people have to tell stories about a series of cartoons featuring a black dog. In one cartoon Blacky defecates between his parents' kennels. Kline (1968) found that people who responded strongly to this cartoon also tended to score high on measures of anal personality traits.

The combined evidence pertinent to the second of our research questions, that there is something truly anal about the anal character, is again somewhat supportive. People who have the traits identified by Freud and his followers as 'anal' do indeed appear to be especially sensitive to things that are dirty, disgusting and faecal. Whether this sensitivity is specifically focused on defecation is unclear, as anal characters seem to have a more general disgust-proneness. However, if we allow anality to include metaphorical filth rather than restricting it to literal faeces then the anal character appears to have been aptly named.

Are anal traits caused by harsh toilet training?

Even if it is true that people with anal traits tend to be preoccupied with or disgusted by matters faecal, it does not follow that toilet-training practices are responsible for those traits. Research on this question has followed two paths, either investigating differences between individuals within one culture or investigating differences between cultures. Studies of the first kind correlate anal traits with the severity of childhood toilet training and studies of the second kind examine the anthropological record to see whether cultural variations in toilet-training practices are associated with culture-wide anal traits.

Researchers who have examined possible associations between the severity of toilet training among children within a particular culture and their later personalities have generally found little support for the Freudian hypothesis. Bernstein (1955) found no tendency for children who had experienced coercive toilet training to be especially likely to collect things, to suffer constipation, or to be unusually fastidious in their finger-painting or on a task requiring them to smear cold-cream. Grinder (1962) found no relationship between the timing or severity of toilet training and resistance to temptation, arguably evidence of orderliness, among 11- and 12-year-old children, and Hetherington and Brackbill (1963) found no correlation between their inventive measures of obstinacy, orderliness and parsimony among 5-year-olds and any dimension of their toilet training, a conclusion also drawn by Sewell et al. (1955).

All of the studies reported to this point examined links between toilet training and personality in childhood. Few have investigated links to adult personality, a more stringent test of Freud's deterministic view of sphincter training. Beloff (1957) failed to find any correlation between anal traits among undergraduates and the toilet-training regimes reported by their mothers. Beloff's study is weakened by its reliance on distant and possibly distorted memories of child-rearing practices. A stronger research design would assess these practices during childhood and examine the children's personalities when they have reached continent adulthood.

This longitudinal approach was taken by McClelland and Pilon (1983), who obtained the only solid evidence for a link between childhood training and adult personality. They found that American 5-year-olds who had experienced more severe toilet training grew up to be 30-year-olds with a relatively high need for achievement. This motive, which drives people towards personal accomplishment, mastery and a sense of control, is not the same thing as the anal character, but resembles some of its more positive facets. However, McClelland and Pilon also found that the adult need for achievement was not uniquely associated with childhood toilet training, but was also linked to other aspects of strict child-rearing such as firm feeding schedules and high parental standards for neatness. In short, it is parental strictness that contributes to the later need for achievement, and severe toilet training is merely one expression of it.

Another set of studies has examined cultural variations in toilet-training practices and their possible effects on personality. Some early anthropological writers did not hesitate to smear whole cultures as essentially anal. Geza Roheim (1934) viewed Western culture, in its preoccupation with hygiene, money and regulations, as completely permeated with anality. The East was not spared, with Gorer (1943) similarly viewing Japanese culture and national character as products of the rigid sphincter training of Japanese infants. Is it indeed the case that cultural variations in anal tendencies are associated with different toilet-training regimes?

The most thorough attempt to examine toilet training and the anal character cross-culturally was conducted by Whiting and Child (1953), who coded anthropological descriptions of a large number of world cultures and also observed the child-rearing methods of a sample of middle-class Chicago residents. The diversity of toilet-training practices was enormous, with some cultures beginning before halfway through the first year of life and others commencing shortly before the age of 5. Severity was also highly variable, some cultures taking a relaxed, gradual and apparently conflict-free approach and others enforcing continence through beatings and public ridicule. However, these cross-cultural variations in the severity of toilet training failed to correlate with variations in other supposedly anal aspects of those cultures. Cultures with harsher toilet training were not especially likely to favour anal explanations for illness, such as seeing diseases as caused by excreta or the failure to dispose of them properly. They had no systematic tendency to employ anal methods of healing, such as prescribing certain forms of elimination or proscribing contact with contaminating substances, and they were not especially guilt-prone. Although none of these findings provide a direct test of whether severe toilet training is associated with anal character traits, they fail to show any hint of such a connection.

Overall, then, there is no compelling evidence for the explanatory role of toilet-training practices in the anal character. Although there may be some suggestive correlations, these are more plausibly explained as side effects of a general link between strict or authoritarian parenting and adult personality, rather than a specific link between the socialization of excretion and the anal triad. As Orlansky (1949) observed, it is a mistake to consider toilet training as an isolated cause of adult personality, when it is part and parcel of the more general approach to socialization that is practised in particular homes and cultures.

On balance, the research literature on Freud's account of the anal character is discouraging. The concept is now moribund, rarely referred to outside the shrinking world of mainstream psychoanalysis. As a topic of psychological research it attracted significant attention in the middle of the twentieth century, a time when psychoanalysis was ascendant within the mental health field, but that attention has dwindled since the 1970s. As a constellation of personality traits, on the other hand, the anal character appears to be real and coherent, and not a mere figment of a theory in decline as some might imagine. More than this, the anal character may have some surprising connections to excrement. Crucially, though, the supposed origin of the anal character in toilet training seems to be simply wrong. Arguably psychoanalysis lost much of its following in modern psychology precisely because of this sort of reductive and deterministic theorizing, where the complexities of adult character could be traced to their messy beginnings in childhood. But in dispensing with the idea of the anal character, has modern personality psychology thrown the baby out with its soiled bathwater?

The return of the anal character

There are reasons to answer this question in the affirmative. The idea of the anal character has not so much disappeared as gone underground, and it has resurfaced in a number of guises. Freed from its psychoanalytic origins and its embarrassing name, this hydra-headed concept lives on in several much better-known psychological ideas, each of which has inspired active and ongoing programmes of research. These ideas differ from classical descriptions of the anal character in many ways – most of them are not merely old wine in new bottles – but they share a family resemblance either with the character type as a whole or with one or more of its component traits.

Obsessive-compulsive personality disorder

The most transparent method of disguise that the anal character has adopted is to transform itself into a mental disorder. Since 1980, the official American system of psychiatric classification, the Diagnostic and Statistical Manual of Mental Disorders (DSM), has recognized a number of disorders of personality, each representing a form of inflexible and maladaptive personality functioning. One of these conditions, obsessive-compulsive personality disorder (OCPD), is strikingly similar to the early psychoanalytic description of the anal character. This connection is not surprising, because the first edition of the DSM, published in 1952, was largely based on a classification developed under the leadership of the famous psychoanalytic psychiatrist William C. Menninger, himself an avid stamp collector (Houts, 2000).

The most recent edition of the DSM (APA, 2000) lists eight features of OCPD which bear a close resemblance to the anal triad. People who receive the diagnosis are likely to be preoccupied with details, rules and lists; to be perfectionistic; and to be excessively devoted to work and productivity, all manifestations of orderliness. Obstinacy is represented by three features: an inflexibly scrupulous morality; rigidity and stubbornness; and a reluctance to delegate tasks to others. Parsimony appears as two final criteria, including miserly spending style and an inability to discard worn-out or worthless objects. To receive an OCPD diagnosis a person need not display the entire triad, requiring only four of the eight features.

OCPD is clinically important because it is one of the more common of the personality disorders, affecting as much as 8 per cent of the general public according to one study (Grant et al., 2004). Levels of OCPD features that do not reach the threshold for diagnosis are more widespread, because although the anal character was initially conceptualized as a discrete personality type it appears to be better understood as a falling on a continuum (Arntz et al., 2009). The disorder affects men and women at similar rates and its onset is thought to be found in childhood, where it can be detected at an early age. The disorder has a large genetic component. Contrary to orthodox Freudian view, there is no evidence that general aspects of the family environment, such as parental strictness or toilet-training philosophy, play any appreciable role in its development (Coolidge et al., 2001; Reichborn-Kjennerud et al., 2007).

Although there is some evidence that personality characteristics that compose the disorder correspond to the three elements of the anal triad (Grilo, 2004), others have argued that its core features are rigidity and perfectionism. These features roughly correspond to the tendency for people with OCPD to have personalities that are closed-minded and conscientious (Lynam & Widiger, 2001). Indeed, there is now strong evidence that OCPD largely represents a maladaptive variant of normal conscientiousness (Samuel & Widiger, 2011). Alternatively, perfectionism can be understood as involving the person's efforts to maintain control of themselves, and rigidity as their stubborn efforts to exert control over others.

The perfectionism of the person with OCPD, their drive to meet high personal standards and their scrupulous attention to detail, may explain why this personality syndrome can be quite functional and highly rewarded, especially in the domain of work. It is one reason why researchers and clinicians sometimes look upon the disorder with some ambivalence, much as Abraham (1923) and Jones (1918/1950) looked upon the anal character. Social value is attached to its traits, but at the extremes they are harmful.

Some of this harm seems to be linked especially to the OCPD person's rigidity. People who are stubborn, who insist on others doing things in their inflexibly preferred ways and who are harsh in their moral judgements, tend to have fraught interpersonal relationships. People with OCPD are especially likely to have poor intimate relations with spouses or partners and may function better in work settings (Costa et al., 2005). Their rigidity has been shown to be associated with explosive outbursts of anger and hostility, and the bearing of grudges (Ansell et al., 2010).

OCPD is important not only as a form of psychopathology in itself, but also as a vulnerability factor for other disorders. There is evidence that it commonly co-occurs with eating disorders and depression, and it may put people at risk of developing them (Costa et al., 2005). Surprisingly, it does not appear to be strongly associated with obsessive-compulsive disorder (OCD), a condition that involves ritualistic behaviours such as washing and checking compulsions and uncontrollable intrusive thoughts, or obsessions. The early psychoanalysts drew no sharp distinction between these two disorders, emphasizing their descriptive similarities, and it appears they were largely wrong to do so.

This brief review of OCPD shows how a thinly disguised version of the anal character has survived the apparent demise of the psychoanalytic concept and found a place within contemporary clinical psychology and psychiatry. The features of this disorder map neatly onto the anal triad, and many of the observations that current writers make about the condition mirror those of Freud, Jones and Abraham a century before. The disorder is widely accepted as a valid form of disturbed personality, and its genetics, its neurobiology and its treatment have been studied extensively. It has made the anal character respectable.

Perfectionism

A preoccupation with things being perfect is an element of the anal character that survives as a diagnostic feature of OCPD. As a normal rather than pathological personality variant perfectionism has also been the subject of an enormous body of research (Flett & Hewitt, 2002). This work tends to see perfectionism as very much a mixed bag. On the one hand, people who strive for perfection for intrinsic reasons and who hold high personal standards tend to function well and cope successfully with the stresses of life. On the other hand, people who have perfectionistic concerns about the discrepancies between their personal expectations and realities, and whose perfectionism is driven by comparisons with others, tend to function poorly and suffer high levels of distress (Stoeber & Otto, 2006). Just as the anal character was viewed ambivalently by early theorists – often productive but joyless – the perfectionist also walks a thin line between sweet success and bitter disappointment.

The idea that there are two distinct forms of perfectionism – variously referred to as functional *vs* dysfunctional, adaptive *vs* maladaptive, normal *vs* neurotic, or healthy *vs* unhealthy – is now very well established. One influential analysis (Frost et al., 1993) proposed that people with the more positive form of perfectionism value order, neatness and organization, have high personal standards that are seen as self-imposed and also hold high standards for others. Studies suggest that this kind of perfectionism is associated with higher levels of well-being, conscientiousness, endurance, achievement and a sense of being in control of one's life (Stoeber & Otto, 2006). People with the more negative form of perfectionism, in contrast, are preoccupied with making mistakes, have doubts about their actions and are therefore indecisive and have standards that they see as prescribed by others, and especially by parents. This form of perfectionism is routinely found to be associated with negative emotional states, stress and burn-out at work. Interestingly, in view of theories of the anal character, people who score high on measures of this form of perfectionism recall their parents as having been relatively harsh. They remember their parents as showing an apparent lack of care and making frequent critical comments, although whether these memories accurately reflect how they were treated in childhood is impossible to assess (Enns et al., 2002).

Whatever its developmental origins and its implications for the well-being of everyday people, perfectionism is strongly associated with a variety of clinical phenomena and mental disorders. Elevated levels of perfectionism are found not only in OCPD, where it is a defining feature, but also in OCD, depression, social anxiety, and eating disorders such as anorexia and bulimia nervosa (Egan et al., 2011). Rather than merely co-occurring with these conditions, perfectionism seems to increase people's risk of developing them and may contribute to maintaining them once they have developed. It can interfere with successful engagement in therapy and be associated with poorer treatment outcomes. Needing to be flawless often gets in the way of becoming merely better, and preoccupation with small flaws can add to the weight of shame, guilt and self-consciousness that bring people into treatment in the first place. In short, perfectionism is a recognizably 'anal' trait that plays a key role in many forms of clinical misery, as well as promoting personal achievement.

Orderliness

The positive form of perfectionism bears a close relationship with orderliness, the first of the three classic anal traits identified by Freud. In his original paper on the anal character, orderliness referred to the tendency to be thorough, reliable, neat, clean and conscientious. It has also been examined extensively in recent personality psychology, which conceptualizes orderliness as a facet of Conscientiousness, one of the five major dimensions of adult personality (McCrae & Costa, 1987). Conscientiousness refers to a broad disposition to be self-controlled, efficient, planful, organized and persevering, and its most recognized facets are Achievement-Striving, Competence, Deliberation, Dutifulness, Order and Self-Discipline. Order in this sense refers to the tendency to be well organized.

Conscientiousness and its facets have been examined in relation to a vast assortment of behaviours, traits and life outcomes. In the previous section of this chapter we saw how the positive form of perfectionism is related to this personality factor. The overwhelming conclusion from existing research is that Conscientiousness-related traits tend to have positive implications. Conscientious people live longer than others (Kern & Friedman, 2008) and orderliness is one of the two facets that is most strongly associated with longevity. Conscientious people tend to be healthier than others, both less vulnerable to common diseases (Goodwin & Friedman, 2006) and more likely to engage in health-promoting behaviour (Bogg & Roberts, 2004). They tend to have more stable marriages (Roberts & Bogg, 2004) and are less prone to divorce (Roberts et al., 2007). In the workplace, Conscientiousness-related traits are the strongest predictors of achievement and career success (Judge et al., 1999). More orderly people tend to perform work tasks at a higher level, although they tend to be weaker when it comes to teamwork and cooperation and less successful in managerial positions (Dudley et al., 2006). In educational settings, more Conscientious students perform better academically and have lower rates of absenteeism and discipline problems (McCann et al., 2009).

Orderliness can also be considered outside the 'Big Five' personality factors as a kind of motivation or need. Preference for order, reflected in a desire for rules and structure, is one facet of the concept of 'need for cognitive closure' (Webster & Kruglanski, 1994). People with high levels of this need seek definite knowledge, make decisions quickly and are bothered by ambiguity. The correlates of need for order include dogmatism, authoritarianism and social prejudice (Van Hiel et al., 2004b).

In sum, the evidence from personality research strongly suggests that the orderliness component of Freud's anal triad has some positive associations, in keeping with the benefits that the early psychoanalysts saw in the trait. However, the scientific evidence again challenges their tracing of anal traits back to toilet training or indeed any aspect of parenting style. Genetic research indicates that Conscientiousness and orderliness are only minimally related to features of the family environment. Much more potent in deciding adults' levels of Conscientiousness are genetic factors and, especially, environmental factors that are unique to the individual rather than shared with his or her siblings (Luciano et al., 2006).

Disgust sensitivity

According to Freud, cleanliness was next to orderliness, not Godliness, and thus a key element of the anal triad. People with anal characters, he argued, were concerned and preoccupied with dirt and hygiene as a reaction formation against their childhood fondness for faeces. By this account, anal characters display an exaggerated disgust response, which enforces their aversion to filth and defends them against an earlier, literal messiness.

As we saw in Chapter 1, disgust has emerged as one of the most fascinating human emotions after a long period of neglect by psychologists. It is an emotion that is at the same time basic, rooted in aversion to disease and decay, and sophisticated, intimately connected to judgements of moral wrongness and impurity. The recent rise of interest in disgust among psychologists has spread to those who study personality. Some people, they observe, are more prone to disgust than others and these differences may be worth studying. They are now referred to as variations in 'disgust sensitivity' (Haidt et al., 1994).

Measures of disgust sensitivity ask people how disgusted they would be to observe things in a number of disgust domains, such as spoiled food, slimy animals, body waste products, mutilation and violations of the body envelope, death, deviant sex and unhygienic practices. There appear to be three underlying facets of disgust sensitivity: 'core disgust', which relates to rejection of offensive stimuli; 'animal reminders', which make us aware of our animal nature and origins; and 'contamination', which relates to the dread of catching a disease or other feared attribute from others.

Excretion features prominently in measures of disgust sensitivity. The most popular brief measure (Olatunji et al., 2007), for example, contains items referring to smelling urine in a railway station tunnel, touching the seat of a public toilet and eating a piece of chocolate shaped like dog faeces. In short, the concept clearly relates to the sort of anxious preoccupations with filth in general, and human excrement in particular, that is one side of the anal character.

The most important thing about disgust sensitivity, however, is not its underlying structure or how it is measured, but the remarkable array of phenomena with which it is associated. People who score higher on disgust sensitivity have a heightened vulnerability to a variety of mental disorders (Olatunji et al., 2009), including hypochondriasis, eating disorders, and phobias of spiders and blood. These phobias are linked to animals and body envelope violations, respectively, suggesting that although they are classified diagnostically as anxiety disorders, they are also, to some extent, disorders of disgust. Intriguingly, disgust sensitivity also confers increased risk for OCD (Tolin et al., 2006), a disturbance in which contamination fears are often prominent and which Freud viewed as closely linked to the anal character.

Disgust sensitivity is associated not only with psychopathology, but also with social attitudes. Disgust-prone people tend to hold more prejudiced views, perhaps especially in relation to homosexuality. For example, Yoel Inbar and colleagues (2009a, b) have shown that disgust-sensitive people are especially likely to have an intuitive or non-conscious disapproval of gays and they are more likely to endorse conservative political views, especially in relation to gay marriage. This link between disgust sensitivity and anti-gay attitudes is interesting because it suggests that disgust rather than fear is the key emotion in what is often but incorrectly referred to as 'homophobia'. It implies that anti-gay prejudice may have some basis in aversion to anal phenomena, based on the association in the popular mind between male homosexuality and the anus.

This link was the basis for one of the most famous studies of cognitive biases, conducted by Loren and Jean Chapman in 1969, which demonstrated how people can observe non-existent or 'illusory' correlations between phenomena when these correlations match their prior expectations. The Chapmans examined responses on the Rorschach inkblot test that were believed by practising psychologists to indicate male homosexuality. They found that psychologists believed responses that identified anal content in blots to be most indicative, although such responses did not, in fact, distinguish homosexual and heterosexual men's Rorschach responses. A plausible basis for the psychologists' mistaken idea was the fact that they strongly associated the concept of homosexuality with anal concepts such as 'rectum' and 'buttocks'.

In a second part of the study, the Chapmans presented non-psychologists with a series of fabricated Rorschach responses that were paired with brief descriptions of the 'emotional problems' that the people who had given them were experiencing. In this series of responses there was no actual correlation between anal Rorschach responses and homosexuality, but the study participants perceived one all the same. Expecting that homosexuality goes with anality, they found (illusory) evidence to support their expectation. We can only guess that the same association underlies the disgust that some people with anti-gay attitudes feel towards gay men.

In addition to its association with prejudice, disgust sensitivity is intimately connected to moral judgements, recalling the psychoanalysts' claims that the anal character is associated with rigid and moralistic standards for behaviour. People who are hypnotically induced to feel disgust express greater moral condemnation for immoral acts (Wheatley & Haidt, 2005), as do people who have been allowed to cleanse their hands with an antiseptic wipe or even those who merely imagine themselves being clean and fresh (Zhong et al., 2010). Findings such as these demonstrate that there is a mental equation of cleanliness and moral purity. Disgust intensifies the judgement that certain people, including the self, are impure. As Freud and others noted in connection with the anal character, disgust-prone people can therefore be rigidly moralistic and harsh in their judgements of those who deviate from social norms.

Authoritarianism

Research on disgust sensitivity shows how personality characteristics associated with the anal character are linked to social attitudes.

Another personality trait that has a strong association with the anal character, and even stronger links to attitudes, is authoritarianism. The psychological study of the authoritarian personality began with the work of Theodor Adorno and his colleagues (1950) who, in the aftermath of World War II and the Holocaust, hoped to lay bare the psychology of anti-Semitism. Their work grew out of an intellectual context in which psychoanalytic ideas about the anal character, obsessional neurosis and the dynamics of paranoia were taken very seriously (Greenstein, 1965). The work soon extended well beyond a search for the underpinnings of hostility to Jews, becoming instead a wide-ranging effort to understand the psychological roots of prejudice and anti-democratic tendencies.

In the course of their research Adorno and his colleagues identified a set of facets of the authoritarian personality, which became the basis for their influential F (for fascism) personality scale. Authoritarians are highly conventional, averse to anything subjective or humanistic, prone to think in rigidly stereotyped ways and uncritically submissive and deferential towards authority figures while being punitive towards subordinates and the weak. Adorno referred to this pattern as the 'bicyclist's personality': 'above they bow, below they kick' (Greenstein, 1965). Authoritarians were also cynical about human nature, likely to see the world as riddled with danger, and they were preoccupied with the sexual lives of others.

Several of these facets resemble aspects of the anal character, particularly the tendency to think in rigid categories, to judge harshly and moralistically people who break the rules and to follow convention in an inflexible manner. Adorno et al. (1950) further claimed that authoritarians tended to be preoccupied with money, neatness, hard work and a view of deviants as 'dirty', all transparently anal descriptions. Their views of the early origins of authoritarian traits are also in keeping with the psychoanalytic theory of the anal character, relating them to overly strict and punishing child-rearing, if not to toilet training in particular.

Later researchers have largely abandoned the F scale and the psychoanalytic accoutrements of Adorno's views on the authoritarian personality that went with it. However, the overlap between authoritarianism and the anal character remains in more recent work. Kline and Cooper (1984) showed that authoritarianism relates to the same underlying dimension of personality as measures of anal or obsessional traits, going so far as to argue that the former is simply the social expression of the latter. Authoritarians have been shown to score high on measures of conscientiousness (Sibley & Duckitt, 2007), compulsiveness (Schlachter & Duckitt, 2002; Van Hiel et al., 2004a), disgust sensitivity (Hodson & Costello, 2007) and need for cognitive closure (Van Hiel et al., 2004b), suggesting that Adorno's psychoanalytically inspired description of the authoritarian character has some empirical foundation.

Meanwhile, modern personality research continues to show that authoritarianism is one of the strongest predictors of social prejudice and endorsement of right-wing ideology. Authoritarianism is strongly related to aversion to a wide variety of groups – racial and sexual minorities, women, immigrants, the mentally ill – and especially towards those who are seen as threatening security and tradition, and those who challenge or oppose mainstream values (Duckitt & Sibley, 2007). In sum, authoritarianism is arguably an attitudinal expression of one element of the anal character. There may be a distinctively anal or obsessional sort of prejudice, as Young-Bruehl (1996) has claimed, which directs its scorn to those who are deviant, dirty and dangerous.

Type A personality

Another relatively modern guise in which the anal character reappears is in ideas of the Type A personality. This supposed personality type, which entered the psychological literature during the 1970s while the anal character was starting to ebb, has achieved fame because of its apparent relationship with ill health (Friedman & Rosenman, 1974). Numerous studies have documented that people with the complex set of traits that compose the type are at an increased risk of coronary heart disease.

Although Type A personality is far from identical to classical descriptions of the anal character, there are some obvious overlaps (Garamoni & Schwartz, 1986). Type A personalities are impatient and have a sense of 'time urgency' that is reminiscent of the concern over the wastage of time that Fenichel (1945) and others related to the anal character's parsimony. The Type A person's overvaluation of money also has its counterpart in the anal character's miserliness. Type A personalities have high levels of hostility and punitiveness, akin to the harshness and 'anal sadism' that Freud remarked on in his original characterization. The fierce devotion to work and productivity that is at the core of Type A personalities is mirrored by the compulsive work ethic and 'Sunday neurosis' of the anal character. Similarly, Type A personalities' strong and somewhat desperate need to be in control, and the perfectionistic personal standards to which they hold themselves, resemble the themes of obstinacy, pathological autonomy, moralistic judgement and rigidity that play such a central role in the anal character's make-up.

As all of these parallels would suggest, measures of Type A personality have been found to correlate well with questionnaires assessing anal and obsessive traits. The correlation is far from perfect, of course, but it reveals some instructive overlaps between Type A behaviour, a form of personality that is recognized as legitimate in contemporary psychology, and an older type that is not.

Collecting and hoarding

In early analyses of the anal triad, parsimony was seen to be at work in frugal and retentive attitudes towards money, in concerns over punctuality and the wasting of time and also in tendencies to collect things. In recent years there has been a small but growing interest in the psychology of collecting and in the related concepts of psychological ownership and attachment to possessions (Pierce et al., 2003). People collect for a variety of reasons, including self-expression, investment, social connection with other collectors, achieving immortality, pure enjoyment of the objects collected and the development of a sense of control or mastery over them. They participate in an often passionate process of setting goals, hunting, acquiring and cataloguing (McIntosh & Schmeichel, 2004), often driven by a desire to assemble a complete and perfect set.

Desires for control, acquisition, classification and perfection fit the anal pattern noted by Ernest Jones, and indeed collectors of this sort have been described as 'taxonomic' to distinguish them from those with more aesthetic motivations (Belk, 1991). Their patterns of collecting are sometimes described as compulsive, addictive or even fetishistic. The only study directly examining the supposed anality of taxonomic collectors, a thesis by Lerner (1961), compared the responses of stamp collectors and non-collectors to 'anally-connotative' words and found that collectors did indeed show the enhanced reaction to them predicted by psychoanalytic theory (Formanek, 1991).

In recent psychology, collecting has been studied less in the context of normal hobbies and more in relation to psychopathology. The pack rat-like hoarding of worthless junk and the unwillingness to throw it away is recognized as one feature of OCPD, the psychiatric legacy of the anal character. In one form, hoarding is a hard-to-treat manifestation of OCD, whose sufferers may feel compelled to amass lint, or whose inability to throw things away may leave them having to squeeze through deep canyons of newsprint in their homes. Hoarding may also occur in the context of other disorders, such as anorexia nervosa or schizophrenia. It appears to have several interrelated dimensions, including living in clutter, being unable to discard things coupled with a strong urge to save them and experiencing strong urges to acquire new things (Frost et al., 2004). In short, hoarders are stingy, strongly attached to possessions and avaricious but disorderly. Their desire for accumulation ultimately defeats their desire for order.

Detail focus

Although Freud's classic description of the anal character did not mention a tendency to focus on fine detail, this narrowing of attention and potential failure to see the forest for the trees has often been taken as a cognitive hallmark of the type. Personality psychologists have approached the concept of detail-orientation from several angles, often under the rubric of 'cognitive style'. Different styles represent habitual ways in which people perceive and interpret their world.

One of the most researched differences in cognitive style is known as field dependence versus independence (Witkin & Goodenough, 1981). Field independent people tend to focus on the distinct features of broader patterns and are adept at extracting elements from their context. This style is often assessed by asking people to discern small figures embedded within a complex visual scene. Field dependent people, in contrast, take a more holistic approach, viewing the elements of the scene within their context and having greater difficulty wrenching the elements from their matrix and seeing them as discrete items. Higher levels of field independence are related to greater personal autonomy but lesser sociability.

A related distinction has been observed when comparing cultures rather than individuals, with social psychologists Richard Nisbett and

Takahiko Masuda (2003) arguing that people in Western cultures tend to have a more 'analytic' style of visual attention, focusing 'locally' on prominent elements of a scene, whereas people from East Asia tend to have a more 'holistic' style, paying greater 'global' attention to the relationships among visual elements and being more sensitive to the surrounding context. For example, Americans tend to zero in on the focal object within an image and describe it as a separate entity, whereas Japanese and Chinese participants tend to direct their gaze to the background of images as well as to the focal object and describe the various elements in relation to one another.

There is some evidence that this sort of detail-focused or analytic cognitive style is indeed associated with other aspects of the anal character. Some researchers have examined individual differences in the processing of visual images that contain conflicting information at the local and global levels. For example, study participants might look at an image of a large letter F that is composed of many small letter Ts. People who score high on a test of field independence attend to the local elements of these images to a greater extent than people who are field dependent: they don't see the F for the Ts (Poirel et al., 2008). Similarly, people with OCPD traits have been shown to pay more attention to the local detail of these compound letters than people without those traits (Yovel et al., 2005). Related to this tendency to focus narrowly on visual detail is a tendency to make narrow conceptual distinctions, a cognitive style known as low 'category width' or 'under-inclusion'. People with OCPD have been shown to categorize words and objects into narrower groupings than other people (Persons & Foa, 1984; Reed, 1985). Once again, we see evidence that one element of the anal character, an excessive focus on detail, is but one part of the broader pattern.

Conclusions

The anal character has fallen from favour as a concept for describing personality. It is tainted by its association with a theoretical approach that is often dismissed as unscientific and of only historical interest. Its very name makes it suspect. As we have seen, however, the personality pattern that the early psychoanalysts brought to light does seem to have some validity, and the elements of that pattern continue to attract the attention of psychologists, even though the pattern itself is rarely acknowledged and the elements have been conceptualized in new ways. The anal character itself has reappeared as OCPD. Orderliness has re-emerged as conscientiousness, perfectionism, disgust sensitivity and detail focus. Obstinacy has come back to scientific life as Type A and authoritarianism, and parsimony has returned as collecting and hoarding.

These many new faces of the anal character are often quite different from one another. They relate to different fields of psychology for a start. OCPD and hoarding are associated with clinical psychology, authoritarianism with social psychology, orderliness with the psychology of personality, Type A with health psychology, and detail focus with cognitive and cultural psychology. These attributes differ in whether they are seen as healthy, like orderliness, pathological, like hoarding and OCPD, or somewhere in between, like perfectionism. They are even somewhat gendered: disgust sensitivity and orderliness being more often apparent in women, and Type A and authoritarianism more common among men. But despite all of these differences of appearance, these anal variants all bear a marked family resemblance.

The anal character has not been consigned to psychology's scrapheap, as we might have thought, but has merely been recycled. Research may have corrected some mistaken ideas about it – the anal type is neither particularly 'anal' in focus, nor is it a true type – and it may have disproven Freud's belief that anal character traits could be traced to the excretory struggles of childhood. But through all of these empirical challenges, the anal character obstinately endures.

6
Potty Mouth

In earlier chapters we examined the psychology of excretion in its solid, liquid and then gaseous forms. It also has an even more ethereal manifestation. Language itself can be filthy – obscene, profane, taboo, vulgar or otherwise offensive. Some of this language is scatological, referring to elimination and its associated body parts. In this chapter we begin by exploring the psychology of swearing, or 'potty mouth', and then turn to a detailed analysis of psychiatric conditions in which it is sometimes taken to extremes. At the close of the chapter we return full circle to solid excrement, examining potty mouth in a more literal and repulsive sense.

The nature of swearing

Defining what counts as swearing is no simple matter, but one linguist proposes four criteria (Ljung, 2011). First, swearing involves the use of taboo words, namely those that are 'too private, too vile or too sacred' (Hughes, 2006, p. 462) to be uttered in polite company. Their taboo quality comes not just from their content, although it is generally off-colour, but also from the form of the word. The same content can often be expressed in a taboo form (*shit*) but also in ways that are scientifically sanitized (*faeces*) or excusably childish (*poo*). Second, the meaning of swear-words is not literal: taboo words draw some of their offensiveness from what they refer to, but they are not used in a way that denotes that meaning. Calling someone an asshole does not involve literally equating the person to the body part, but expresses the speaker's denigrating attitude. Third, swearing tends to be formulaic, employing a few established expressions in inflexible and uncreative ways. Finally, swearing is emotive: it usually accompanies and expresses strong and abrupt emotions, most often anger but also surprise, dismay, pain, disappointment, fear and even sudden happiness.

Swearing does many kinds of linguistic work. It often involves sudden exclamations, known as 'expletive interjections' (*Bugger!*), and also occurs in oaths (*By God!*) and emphatic denials (*My arse I will!*). Frequently swearing expresses the speaker's ill-will towards a hearer, including curses (*To hell with you!*), ritual insults (*Your mother is a whore!*), expletive epithets (*Wanker!*) and what one linguist delicately calls 'unfriendly suggestions' (*Get fucked!*) (Ljung, 2011). Some swearing takes place merely as a slot-filler, adding intensity and emotional bite to the expression that surrounds it (*Not bloody likely!*).

In addition to these differences in linguistic form, swearing can be classified on the basis of its content. Profanity is swearing that uses religious terms in a way that may be offensive to believers but that is not intended as a challenge to their beliefs. Blasphemous swearing occurs when the speaker is deliberately challenging religious beliefs and symbols. Obscenity includes swearing with sexual content, whereas vulgarity refers to swearing that extends beyond the sexual realm to include other body parts and functions.

These distinctions point to the existence of a limited number of common themes in swearing. Some taboo words and expressions have religious or supernatural content, referring either to good and heavenly things (*God*) or to diabolical ones (*damn*). Another theme is made up of offensive animal terms. Some taboo words are sexual, referring to particular organs or acts. Scatological words refer to the products, processes and body parts involved in excretion. Slurs are taboo terms for ethnic groups, genders or sexual minorities. Other popular themes include terms and expressions referring to mothers, illegitimacy, illnesses and death. Different themes may also combine into a single taboo expression: *goddamn son of a bitch* contains celestial and diabolical content, a gender slur, an animal term and a statement about motherhood.

Scatological swearing

Evidently, although taboo language is sometimes referred to as 'potty mouth', its content is not narrowly excremental. The use of a toilet metaphor to describe this diverse assortment of expressions merely indicates that taboo language is seen as symbolically dirty. 'Potty mouth' reveals how excrement serves as the prototype of filth, even if scatological language is only one of the many kinds of swearing.

Even so, scatological terms appear to be particularly central to swearing. According to one systematic review of swearing in 25 languages, 'scatology is the undisputed leader among the taboo themes used in… expletive epithets' (Ljung, 2011, p. 135). Coining the useful term 'faecalia' to refer to these expressions, Ljung observes that scatological terms are among the most popular expletive epithets in English, with *arsehole* or *asshole, fart, prat, shit* and *turd* especially common. Another group of sodomy-related epithets (e.g., *bugger, sod*) also has an anal theme but is not usually considered scatological. The scatological lexicon is tilted heavily towards faecal and to a lesser extent flatulent terms, with urinary words less numerous, less frequently used, less offensive and less linguistically flexible: *piss* is not used as an epithet or expletive interjection, but only in so-called 'destinational' expressions (*piss off*) and indirectly to refer to the state of being drunk or, in the USA, angry (*pissed*). Just as faeces is more disgusting and contaminating than urine, *shit* is more offensive than *piss*.

Shit is consistently among the two most frequently uttered swearwords in English and can be used in a bewildering variety of ways. Kipfer and Chapman's (2007) helpful dictionary of American slang lists eight non-literal meanings of the noun – nonsense, disrespect, things of inferior quality, possessions, an obnoxious person, drugs, nothing and misfortune – and two meanings of the verb form (to lie or to respond with powerful emotion). The adjective *shitty* is also semantically versatile, labelling things as nasty, tedious or unwell. *Shit* joins promiscuously with other words to convey an enormous range of meanings. These may reference states of mind such as anger (*shit-a-brick*), fright (*shit-scared* or *scared shitless*), surprise (*no shit!*), mockery (*tough shit*) or intoxication (*shit-faced*). They may also convey a range of evaluations of people: that they are successful (*shit-hot*), stupid (*shit-for-brains*), mistaken (*full of shit*), insignificant (*shit-ass*), depraved (*shit-heel*), smug (*shit-eating grin*), sanctimonious (*believe one's shit doesn't stink*), rural (*shit-kicker*) or young (*shitty-britches*). Kindred expressions extend the range from the boastful (*crapper*) to the obsequious (*brown-noser*).

Scatological swearing is by no means confined to the English language, however, and takes inventive and original forms in many others (Ljung, 2011). Spaniards utter the expletive *Me cago en Dios* (I shit on God) and Arabs may curse *khara alaik* (may there be shit on you). There is an especially rich trove of scatological epithets and insults. Afrikaans has *gatkruiper* (arse-creeper), Cantonese has *sí fat gwái* (asshole ghost), Finnish has *kusipää* (pisshead) and Russian has *govnó* (shit-eater). Animal combinations figure in the Greek *kopróskilo* (shit dog), the Mandarin *gǒu-pì* (dog fart) and a Central African expression meaning 'Your mouth is as flabby as the arse of an elephant.' Scatological language appears to be universal: as Ljung argues, it is 'a feature of all languages that vernacular words denoting excrement are among the first to be adopted as swear words' (p. 67).

This introduction can only begin to sketch the richness and complexity of taboo language. Many historical, linguistic and cultural studies have been devoted to this pungent topic, emphasizing the origins of swear-words, the complexities of their syntax and semantics – such as why it is grammatical to say 'two loaves of bread' but not 'two turds of shit' – and the uses of obscenity in sexual harassment and social interaction (e.g., Dooling, 1996; Hughes, 1991; Ljung, 2011; McEnery, 2005; Montagu, 1967). In contrast, there has been relatively little research of a psychological nature, with the notable exception of Timothy Jay's work (e.g., 1992, 2000). Even so, we now know a good deal about bad language.

Who swears (and who cares)?

One of the key psychological questions in the study of swearing is whether some people swear more than others. For example, do people with some personality characteristics swear excessively and those with others show greater than average restraint? Jay (2000) speculates that people with antisocial or Type A personalities, who are impatient, competitively driven and often volcanically hostile, are especially avid swearers, but there has been little research to confirm these guesses. There is some unsurprising evidence that religious people are less disposed to swear: one study of secondary school students finding that those from a religious school were slower to utter taboo sexual words projected onto a screen (Grosser & Laczek, 1963). Whether this apparent suppression extended from the formal setting of the testing room to the playground was not examined. More religious people may not only swear less, but also appear to be more offended by it (Wober, 1990).

One reason often given for the greater linguistic decorum of religious people is guilt or anxiety surrounding taboo activities such as sex. It is often asserted that people who suppress something in themselves, and urge others to do likewise, have conflicts or 'hang-ups' about it. One interesting study of the use of taboo language can be seen in this light (Motley & Camden, 1985). Male participants were given a task in which they had to select an ending for a series of incomplete sentences from a set of four options. One of the options involved a sexual double entendre (e.g., 'The old hillbilly liked to keep his moonshine in big…' 1) jugs, 2) bottles, 3) cauldrons, or 4) vats). The task was administered by a female experimenter described as 'sexually provocative in attire and behaviour [albeit] within the extreme limits of what might reasonably be expected in a laboratory situation' (p. 128). In these arousing conditions, men who had high levels of sexual guilt were much more likely than others to chose the sexually suggestive options. By implication, people who have strict moral qualms about sexual impropriety might be especially drawn to offensive language and ideas, even if they may be unlikely to express them.

Swearing may be related to mental disorder as well as personality. Some recent research finds that swearing may sometimes be an indicator of emotional distress among young people. One study showed that vicious cursing and foul language were strongly associated with making suicide threats among children and adolescents with bipolar disorder (Papolos et al., 2005). Another study found that adolescents who used more swear-words when describing their personality in a blog entry tended to be more depressed and were also judged to be more depressed by readers who did not know them (Rodriguez et al., 2010). Use of swear-words was more strongly associated with writers' levels of depression than their use of words related to sadness and death, or their non-use of words referring to positive emotions. In short, online swearing was a highly sensitive index of depressive misery. Interestingly, swear-words were not associated with depression when people wrote personality self-descriptions in a private diary, implying that it is only when swearing is used to communicate with others that it reveals the person's unhappiness.

Swearing features in another mental disorder in a more directly communicative way. 'Telephone scatologia', in which people compulsively make obscene phone calls to strangers, is considered a form of 'paraphilia' or perversion. Like exhibitionists, people with this condition are sexually gratified by making lewd but touch-free contact with their victims, and part of their gratification comes from the shock and fear that they provoke. The condition has been conceptualized as a 'courtship disorder' (Freund & Blanchard, 1986) as it involves an apparent difficulty or fixation at one phase in the process of acquiring a mate. Stuck in this 'pretactile interaction' stage, people with the condition may lack the social confidence to go further, or simply prefer the anonymity of the encounter.

Telephone scatologia may be associated with other difficulties, including antisocial personality traits, low intelligence, social isolation and other sexual deviations, but sometimes at least the sense of humour remains intact. One telephone scatologist, facing a harassment charge in court, asked the judge how many perverts and felons were on the jury. When told that there were none he objected, arguing that he was supposed to be judged by his peers (Pakhomou, 2006).

Swearing and gender

One factor that influences people's propensity to swear is gender. Swearing is a stereotypically masculine activity, some arguing that it is part of men's brute biology: 'men swear because we are uncouth warthogs by nature' (Dooling, 1996, p. 5). Alternatively, gender differences in swearing may reflect nurture and the different social expectations that govern men's and women's speech. We can approach the link between gender and swearing from three angles. Do women or men produce more swearing, do they perceive it differently and are they the targets of it in different ways?

It is well documented that men tend to swear more than women (Jay & Janschewitz, 2008). Men also tend to use more offensive swear-words and to employ a wider array (Jay & Janschewitz, 2008). These findings create a small paradox, because people tend to associate swearing with being in positions of low status and power (Jay, 1992), and men are less likely to hold these positions. A possible solution to this paradox is that men's swearing sometimes reflects an attempt to achieve identity and status within same-sex groups. Men sometimes seek this kind of 'covert prestige' – a form of status that involves embracing blue-collar authenticity – by using coarse and confrontational language, as if linguistic propriety were a feminine quality to be avoided at all costs. Rougher forms of speech express male identity, solidarity and physical power (Kiesling, 1998).

The importance of gendered groups for swearing can be seen clearly in findings that both men and women swear more in same-sex company (Jay, 1992; Wells, 1989), showing more restraint in mixed settings. Choice of terms may also become more delicate in mixed company. A study conducted in 1979 found that men's preferred copulatory term was 'fucking' when speaking to men and 'screw' when speaking to a mixed audience, whereas women preferred 'screw' in the same-sex environment and 'make love' when men were present (Jay, 2000).

Women and men may also differ in how they perceive the use of taboo language. Women tend to judge swearing to be more offensive and swear-words to be more powerful (Dewaele, 2004). Although it has been argued that girls are socialized against swearing more strongly than boys – that 'If a little girl "talks rough" like a boy, she will be ostracized' (Lakoff, 1975, p. 5) – no such difference in punishment was recalled recently by female and male university students (Jay et al., 2006). In the present time, when differences in the perceived acceptability of male and female swearing are dwindling, it is more likely that women judge swearing more negatively for reasons other than a socialized double standard. Possibly, they are more likely to view verbal aggression as endangering interpersonal relationships (Jay & Janschewitz, 2008).

In addition to differences in how men and women produce and perceive swearing, there are differences in the taboo language that targets them. Terms of abuse that refer to excrement, masturbation and being cuckolded tend to target men, whereas women are more likely to be the targets of taboo animal terms, such as *bitch* and *cow* (Hughes, 1991; Van Oudenhoven et al., 2008). Animal expressions are also seen as especially offensive when directed towards women (Haslam et al., 2011).

Why this might be so is a fascinating question. There is a long history of animal metaphors being used to refer to women – from endearing pet names to terms of abuse – and many continue to this day, including some that are not invariably seen as taboo, such as *chick*, *filly*, *fox* and *kitten*. The metaphorical closeness of women and animals may reflect the ancient belief that women are closer to nature than men (Ortner, 1972). This link survives to the present day: people tend to mentally associate women with nature, and media images tend to picture women in the context of nature more than men (Reynolds & Haslam, 2011). Sexuality is also involved in the link. One study showed that when women are pictured in objectified ways, half-naked and sexually provocative, they are associated more with animal-related words ('nature', 'hibernation', 'instinct', 'paw', 'snout') than are unobjectified women or men, whether objectified or not (Vaes et al., 2011). The fact that women are more often targets of taboo animal terms reveals a deeper, lingering association between women and beasts.

Swearing and culture

As a linguistic and symbolic phenomenon it should come as no surprise that swearing and cursing vary across cultures. People from different language communities have different sets of taboo words and these sets may reveal different preoccupations. In highly religious communities blasphemous terms may be the most taboo, and in those where machismo dominates, insults referring to male homosexuality and effeminacy may be especially potent and common. In principle it should be possible to learn something important about a culture from how it swears and from the words it taboos.

There have been disappointingly few psychological studies of cross-cultural variations in swearing. One interesting exception is a study comparing preferred terms of abuse in the north and south of Italy (Semin & Rubini, 1990). Although the language of these regions is essentially the same, people from the industrialized north tend to hold more individualist values, believing strongly in personal achievement and self-reliance. Those from the south have a reputation for more collectivist values, in which the good of the family and community comes before the good of the individual, and people acquire their identities from belonging to these groups. If the values of people from north and south differ, then the insults they prefer to use may illuminate those differences. Indeed they did. Insults from the north tended to cast aspersions on the personal qualities of individuals, whereas those of southerners tended to challenge the reputation of entire families. Typical northern insults, for example, referred to their target's stupidity, ugliness and lack of manners, and also used a variety of animal, sexual and excremental terms. In contrast, southern insults more often focused on the target's relationships, declaring incestuous attachments to mothers, homosexuality of fathers, animal parentage of sisters and death wishes against kin. A classic example was 'Fuck off you and 36 of your relatives.'

A more extensive cross-cultural study of terms of abuse was conducted by van Oudenhoven et al. (2008), who recruited participants from 11 European nations, the USA and Canada. Study participants were asked what they would say to someone who rudely bumped into them without apology. Several distinctive patterns emerged. Devil-related expressions were unusually prominent in Norway, genital terms in Croatia and France, and mental abnormality or stupidity in Italy, Spain and Greece. Abuse related to the anal zone was especially prominent in Germany and the USA, although scatological expressions were also among the five most commonly chosen terms of abuse in France and Italy. The authors argue that the German preference for anal terms of abuse reflects a cultural value placed on cleanliness. Their speculation accords with the controversial work of folklorist Alan Dundes (1984), who discerned a pattern of supposedly anal themes in German folktales, slang, profanity, jokes and musical tastes (i.e., preference for the sound of wind instruments).

Being rudely bumped features in another fascinating study of culture and swearing. Focusing on responses to being sworn at rather than the swearing lexicon, Dov Cohen and colleagues (1996) examined how men from the southern and northern states of the USA reacted to being bumped and called an 'asshole'. Theorizing that the American South has a 'culture of honour', in which slights against one's dignity and manhood must be avenged, the researchers predicted that southerners but not northerners would react angrily and aggressively to the insult. As they expected, men from southern states were more likely to think that their masculine reputation had been challenged, secreted more stress hormones and testosterone, indicating emotional upset and preparation for angry retaliation, and were subsequently more likely to act in an aggressive or dominant manner. As this work shows, cultural variations can be seen in the production of swearing and also in how it is perceived.

Functions of swearing

Why do people swear and curse? Many kinds of answer are possible, but three stand out. First, people might swear primarily to express themselves; that is, we might swear to give spoken form to what we feel and think, including what we think about who we are. Second, people might swear as a way of communicating. Whereas expressing oneself does not require an audience and its goal is to put one's mind into words, communication involves an attempt to influence other people's minds. A third answer to the puzzle of why we swear involves self-regulation: people might use swearing, apparently an out-of-control behaviour, as a way to manage and influence their own emotions and actions. Swearing might be functional as a way of helping us achieve control over ourselves rather than as a way of losing it.

The idea that swearing is primarily expressive is intuitively appealing. Expletives seem to be mindless and almost reflex-like, emitted too quickly and automatically to be deliberate attempts to communicate with others. They are sometimes uttered when no one else is in earshot. Swearing often seems to involve a venting of emotion which serves the beneficial function of releasing anger and displeasure. According to one writer, it 'achieves the same catharsis one gets from a hearty belch... it's a psychic purgative when one is suffering from emotional constipation' (Dooling, 1996, p. 8).

For all its commonsense appeal, psychological evidence for this sort of catharsis is flimsy. Rather than draining away anger, expressions of hostility are more likely to sustain it (Bushman, 2002). Venting anger tends to maintain the person's sense of being wronged than it is to relieve it, and thus more likely to lead to aggressive behaviour. Although people tend to think of anger as a toxic quantity that should not be 'bottled up', a better metaphor may be the fire that should not be stoked. Often doing nothing or seeking distractions is better than trying to vent and the same may go for expletive swearing. It may express our anger and annoyance, but it is unlikely to reduce them.

Whether or not swearing is an effective form of expression, it is clearly an effective form of communication. By swearing, especially in its more deliberate rather than expletive forms, people are aiming to influence others. Sometimes what is being communicated is hostility, so that the hearer recognizes the speaker's emotion and responds appropriately, apologizing, avoiding or confronting as the case may be. Swearing adds intensity to an emotional message and also implies that the speaker is at least momentarily uninhibited and thus capable of acting aggressively. Because angry swearing can produce submissive responses it can sometimes be used deliberately to produce them, even when the speaker is not genuinely angry. This calculated use of swearing is an instrumental attempt to intimidate others, making it a valuable part of the repertoire of bullies and harassers. At other times what is being communicated by swearing is just a desire for attention: by violating polite rules of speech, people, and especially young ones, can get noticed by others.

Still another way in which swearing communicates is by demonstrating that the swearer belongs to a group. In this way, swearing communicates a sense of shared identity. The phenomenon of 'covert prestige' is a case in point, where men deliberately adopt rough styles of speech, especially when speaking with one another, precisely because they are seen as incorrect and low-status. Swearing among men can communicate a sense of being part of a masculine group, untamed and rebellious.

Compared to the view that swearing expresses emotion or communicates identity, the idea that it might also be something we use to regulate ourselves sounds dubious. We are accustomed to thinking of swearing as something done impulsively in the grip of strong emotion or as a way of influencing others, not as a deliberate attempt to influence oneself. Nevertheless, one study suggests that swearing may serve a useful self-regulating function when it comes to pain control (Stephens et al., 2009). English undergraduates were asked to immerse their hands in icy water for as long as they could stand – a standard laboratory test of pain tolerance – either while repeating a swear-word of their choice or, in the control condition, while repeating an inoffensive neutral word. Not only did participants keep their hands immersed about 35 per cent longer while swearing than while intoning the neutral word, but their heart rate also increased more and they perceived their pain to be milder. The researchers concluded that swearing induces a negative emotional state, most probably aggressive, which promotes a fight or flight response. This activated bodily response enables people to not merely tolerate pain but to dull the experience of it. Although the idea has yet to be tested, people in pain might swear as either an intentional or a learned but unconscious tactic for dulling its intensity.

We can speculate on additional possibilities. People may use dirty language in sexual contexts not just to shock or titillate a partner but also to increase or maintain their own arousal, as appears to be the case in telephone scatologia. They may swear at umpires and referees not just to express anger or communicate hostility but also to fuel and prolong their righteous indignation, one of the most enjoyable of emotions. They may curse their predicament during a long and tedious activity in a semi-deliberate effort to bolster their drive and energy. In short, swearing serves a variety of purposes: expression, communication and self-management.

Coprolalia

Filthy language takes a particularly pathological form in Gilles de la Tourette's syndrome, a condition in which people are afflicted by involuntary actions called tics. Motor tics can include grimacing, twitching, blinking, finger sniffing, joint cracking, tongue poking, head tossing and a variety of contortions and awkward motions of the body. Vocal tics can include grunts, barks, yelps and the repetition of what has just been heard ('echolalia'). Perhaps the best-known kind of vocal tic, although in fact it is only found in a minority of people with Tourette's syndrome, is the uncontrollable blurting of obscenities, or 'coprolalia'. Unlike telephone scatologia, where obscene speech is a deliberate attempt to arouse the speaker and shock the hearer, coprolalia is involuntary.

Coprolalia was present in one of the first recorded cases of Tourette's syndrome. The Marquise de Dampierre, a young woman described as having 'distinguished manners', would suddenly exclaim 'shit and fucking pig' at inopportune and embarrassing times. The French physician Jean Itard, who reported her case in 1825, did not treat the Marquise, but made pioneering efforts to assist other sufferers reported in his original paper (Kushner, 1999). His preferred treatments included chicken soup, long baths and leeches applied to the genitals.

Although coprolalia strictly means 'shit speech' its content is not limited to excremental words and includes profane and sexual language, animal names and racial slurs. Some of the more colourful examples include *eingeschlagene schaedeldecke* ('smashed skull' in German) and a Peruvian who repeatedly exclaimed 'serve me coffee' (Van Lancker & Cummings, 1999). Less frequently, Touretters may also perform obscene actions such as making sexual gestures (copropraxia) or writing obscene material (coprographia) (Freeman et al., 2009). They may also use language that is not obscene but merely socially inappropriate, such as blurting out insults. One study found that almost a quarter of Tourette's syndrome patients habitually insulted others, focusing most often on their weight, intelligence, appearance and breath or body odour. A larger proportion reported having urges to insult others and needing to suppress them (Kurlan et al., 1996). Despite this diversity of forms, all of these coprophenomena have in common a capacity to offend others.

Coprolalia and related phenomena may be filthy in a general rather than narrowly excremental sense, but excretion-related words feature prominently, consistent with their primal and taboo nature. The original case of the Marquise bears this out and other early cases reported by Gilles de la Tourette himself were equally faecal in content: one 12-year-old boy shouting 'shitty asshole' and a 15-year-old boy shouting what Tourette euphemistically referred to as 'the word of Cambronne', a general under Napoleon who at the Battle of Waterloo is reputed to have said 'Merde!' when invited to surrender by the British.

Similar content dominates the case of Wolfgang Amadeus Mozart, a coprographic as much as a musical prodigy (Simkin, 1992). His letters contain a rich trove of excretory terminology: in decreasing order of frequency they refer to buttocks and defecation, shit, arse, muck, piddle or piss, fart and arse hole, and make reference to such make-believe characters as Duchess Smackbottom, Countess Makewater and Princess Dunghill. He was also given to singing or reciting vulgar rhymes about 'muck, shitting and arse-licking'. Whether Mozart's writing and speech were uncontrollable and tic-like rather than deliberately perverse and puerile is difficult to say.

Research on contemporary coprolalia confirms that excremental language is still dominant. A review of common coprolalic utterances in six countries (Singer, 1997) finds excretion-related words in five of them. In addition to the familiar *shit, ass(hole)* and *piss* of the Anglo-Saxon countries, we have the more exotic Danish *gylle* (animal faeces) and the unique Japanese expression *kusobaba* (shit grandma). One deaf person with coprolalia repeatedly 'blurted' shit in American Sign Language (Lang et al., 1993).

Coprolalia seems to cry out for psychological explanation because it is clearly meaningful: Touretters do not blurt out random or innocuous words. It sometimes displays a kind of mischievous intelligence, as if calculated to cause maximum offence in a particular social setting. One patient, for example, falsely confessed to a murder when police came to his door for routine questioning of neighbourhood residents and reported 'an urge to say exactly the most inappropriate comment possible' in many settings (Kurlan et al., 1996). Coprolalia also seems meaningful because it dramatizes the idea of psychological conflict, the timeless battle between impulse and self-control. People with Tourette's syndrome wish they did not utter obscenities, feel ashamed and embarrassed that they do and often try valiantly to suppress and disguise their vulgar speech. One sufferer reached out with his hand immediately after shouting obscenities in an effort to 'catch the word and bring it back before others can hear it' (Jankovic, 2007). Others camouflage their vocal tics by altering speech sounds, muttering the obscenities or even saying them silently ('mental coprolalia').

Early writers developed a variety of accounts of the psychological causation of Tourette's syndrome. Sigmund Freud proposed that 'convulsive tics' were closely related to the phenomenon of hysteria, the condition that was the proving ground for his new therapeutic method of psychoanalysis. One of his hysterical patients, Frau Emmy von N., suffered from an assortment of tics including 'clacking' sounds and facial contortions. The Hungarian psychoanalyst Sandor Ferenczi argued that tics derived from the repression of masturbatory impulses – 'eruptive cursing' was a symbolic expression of erotic desires – an ironic reversal of an earlier theory that held the expression of these impulses responsible for producing tics (Kushner, 1999).

More recently, theorists have considered complex tics, such as coprolalia, to be equivalent to the compulsions found in obsessive-compulsive disorder (OCD), a condition whose psychological dimension is well established. Although in theory compulsions are more voluntary than tics – they are deliberately performed in response to a strong inner pressure to act rather than being involuntary – in practice the boundary between them is blurred. Tourette's syndrome and OCD commonly occur together and increasingly they are seen as falling on a single psychiatric spectrum.

The idea that Tourette's syndrome in general and coprolalia in particular are psychologically meaningful is hard to shake, but evidence that it has a primarily biological origin is also very strong. The syndrome has a very strong genetic component: if one identical twin suffers from it there is an 89 per cent chance that his or her co-twin will also be affected, rising to 100 per cent if the milder but related 'chronic multiple tic disorder' is considered as well (Singer, 2000). Purely neurological causes can precipitate Tourette's syndrome, such as carbon monoxide poisoning, streptococcal brain infections and even wasp stings. Similarly, coprolalia can be observed in other clinical conditions besides Tourette's syndrome that have a plainly neurological basis, such as frontotemporal dementia, as well as after injuries to the brain following encephalitis and stroke.

Neuroscientific research increasingly indicates that Tourette's syndrome is associated with anatomical and physiological abnormalities in such brain regions as the basal ganglia, caudate nuclei and the frontal cortex (Jankovic, 2007). Tics also respond well to medical treatments and in particular to a variety of antipsychotic, antidepressant or tranquillizing medications. Despite all this evidence of biological causation, the syndrome may sometime emerge in response to life experiences. One Saudi Arabian girl, for instance, developed coprolalia, facial tics and compulsive spitting shortly after being severely frightened by a group of cockroaches in a dark toilet (el-Assra, 1987).

How do we square the apparent meaningfulness and psychological richness of coprolalia with the evidence that it is primarily a reflection of genetic and neurological abnormalities? The most promising explanation is that Tourette's syndrome is primarily a disorder of defective inhibition and impulse control. The brain regions and neurophysiological systems implicated in the syndrome enable executive control of action, including the inhibition of behaviour that is judged ill-advised, dangerous or socially inappropriate. Symptoms such as the blurting of obscenities and the failure to suppress unusual movements reflect this lack of behavioural inhibition and so do several of the associated features of the syndrome. Sufferers are frequently troubled by problems with attention and concentration, commonly receiving diagnoses of attention deficit hyperactivity disorder (ADHD). They sometimes have difficulties with sexually inappropriate behaviour and anger control, and may be prone to outbursts of violence and self-injury. All of this implies a fairly general inability to inhibit action.

Coprolalia therefore seems to be best explained as a neurologically based failure to stifle impulses to say and do offensive things. What makes those things offensive, and hence deserving of inhibition, depends on human psychology and culture. For this reason, the blurted speech of coprolalic patients always has taboo content, both excremental and sexual, and ideas or expressions that are particularly offensive in a particular culture, such as 'shit grandma' for the elder-respecting Japanese, will feature prominently in that culture's coprolalic lexicon. Consequently, coprolalia is psychologically revealing even if it is not psychologically caused. The failure of Touretters to inhibit their impulses to say dirty things is not caused by an inner conflict or a perverse desire to offend others, but reflects a sort of brake failure in the brain. Like all of us, people with Tourette's syndrome experience conflict between their impulses and their wishes not to behave badly, but that conflict is more visible (and audible) in them because the battle between impulse and inhibition is less evenly matched than it is for the rest of us.

Even if Tourette's syndrome is primarily biological in origin, it may still respond to psychological treatments. Some of the behavioural techniques that have demonstrated effectiveness include massed practice, in which the patient is instructed to deliberately and repetitively perform the tic, and habit reversal training, in which patients re-enact the tic in front of a mirror to gain increased awareness of the tics, identify situations where the risk of tics is particularly high and train themselves to carry out behaviours that negate tics (Jankovic, 2007). By implication, coprolalics might paradoxically be well advised to increase their cursing, but to do so in a more deliberate, earnest and reflective manner.

Coprophagia

Coprolalia has a rather indirect link to excrement. The content of the blurted obscenities of Tourette's patients is not restricted to excretion and it is expressed symbolically as taboo words. In coprophagia, or 'shit eating', the link is disgustingly literal. This is 'potty mouth' in a non-metaphorical sense, although it must be noted that one writer has seen a metaphorical link between coprophagia and the apparently innocent act of reading (Strachey, 1930).

Although eating excrement might seem to be so profoundly contrary to instinct that it should occur rarely if ever, it is surprisingly common. It can of course occur inadvertently, this being a major source of parasitic infections in humans, such as the hookworm infestations in the American South that may be responsible for the association of 'poor white trash' with filth in the public imagination (Wray, 2006). However, it can also occur quite deliberately. As Rozin and Fallon (1987) show, humans have no innate aversion to excrement and only come to acquire a revulsion in early childhood. Children younger than 3, for example, show positive responses to faecal odours and in one study a majority of 2-year-olds put imitation dog faeces (artfully crafted from smelly cheese and peanut butter) in their mouths when it was offered to them on a plate (Rozin et al., 1986).

Coprophagic tendencies are also widespread among non-human animals. Many insects, such as the dung beetle, use the excrement of other creatures as a food source. For rabbits and rodents, eating excrement has a nutritional purpose, enabling the complete digestion of complex carbohydrates. Elephants reportedly feed their dung to their calves, apparently to ensure that they acquire the intestinal flora necessary for digestion. Our close evolutionary cousins the pygmy chimpanzees or bonobos have been observed inspecting and then eating their excrement, possibly because a first passage through the digestive system softens hard seeds that can otherwise not be broken down (Sakamaki, 2010). The coprophagic behaviour of captive animals may sometimes be an indicator of stress, boredom and nutrient or roughage deficiency, and minimizing it is a frequent concern of farmers, veterinarians and zoo-keepers.

Among humans, coprophagia sometimes occurs in the context of pica, a disorder typically observed in childhood in which people eat non-food substances. In addition to faeces, common substances include paint, hair, paper and soil. In young children and intellectually disabled adults this pattern of eating inappropriate substances is often relatively indiscriminate and opportunistic, scavenging whatever is at hand that is small enough to fit into the mouth. Needless to say this behaviour carries potentially serious health risks, including infectious disease, parasites, intestinal obstruction and poisoning, as when children eat chips of lead-based paint. Intriguingly, pica among intellectually disabled adults appears to be strongly associated with a lack of supportive relationships and social contact with family members (Ashworth et al., 2009). Is it too much to infer that pica sufferers are, in part, hungry for love?

Occasionally pica emerges in adulthood among people without intellectual disability and has a compulsive and highly selective quality: the patient feels an overwhelming craving for a particular kind of substance. One case in point is a young woman with anorexia nervosa who developed a pattern of compulsive toilet-paper eating (Yalug et al., 2007). This patient's paper-eating may have played a role in maintaining or even causing her eating disorder, as the ingested paper would induce feelings of fullness without providing calories. Similarly compulsive in nature is the case of a 17-year-old Ethiopean woman who developed a compulsion to eat a mud wall in front of her house. At the time she presented for treatment she suffered from severe abdominal distension, constipation and pain, having eaten 8 square metres of the wall (Baheretibeb et al., 2008). Troubled by intrusive thoughts and images of eating the mud whenever she left home, she would descend on it 'greedily' when she returned. These two cases suggest that in some instances pica can be akin to OCD.

Turning from pica in general to coprophagia in particular, we can see that a single behaviour can have a multitude of causes. Coprophagia is most commonly observed in intellectually disabled children and adults, and even in this group there can be a diversity of motivations. Sometimes, especially when it is accompanied by other off-putting toileting behaviour such as 'rectal digging' and 'faecal smearing', it seems to be merely chaotic. At other times coprophagic behaviour may be motivated by the attention it receives, as episodes of coprophagia are typically followed by tender bodily attention from caregivers (Beck & Frohberg, 2005; Schroeder, 1989). Yet another dynamic was at work in the case of a man with profound developmental disabilities, who appeared to find the smell and taste of his own faeces appealing and ate them for self-stimulation (Baker et al., 2005). His psychologists were able to eliminate his coprophagic episodes simply by spicing up the man's diet, adding curry dishes to his menu and making peppery and pungent snacks available between meals. His unsavoury habit appears to have been a response to an unsavoury diet.

Coprophagia is sometimes observed among older adults suffering from dementia, in whom diffuse brain damage may lead to a loss of normal inhibitions. It has been suggested that the behaviour may arise as a way to conceal faecal incontinence (Ghaziuddin & McDonald, 1985) or as a regression to infantile oral habits (Arieti, 1944). In the latter case, the coprophagic behaviour of demented adults is akin to the behaviour of small children who have yet to learn the normal disgust reaction to faeces, or to the behaviour of intellectually disabled people who have failed to learn it. Whatever its causes in this population, the behaviour can have fatal consequences among the elderly such as choking (Byard, 2001) and it is hard to imagine anything that could more tragically rob the dignity of people in their final years of life.

The eating of faeces occurs infrequently in response to psychotic delusions and auditory or visual hallucinations. Coprophagia may occur in obedience to commanding voices (Chaturvedi, 1988) or in accordance with a system of delusional beliefs. For example, one elderly psychotic woman ate her own faeces and drank her urine in the belief that this revitalized her, and would pour her recycled urine, mixed with lemon syrup and fruit, into holes drilled in trees as a way to infuse them with her life (McGee & Gutheil, 1989). Another delusional man carried out the same eating behaviours from a conviction that his bodily excretions and secretions – also including earwax and nasal mucus – had to be preserved (Razali, 1998). Although coprophagia can be treated with anti-psychotic medications in cases like these (Harada et al., 2006), in the latter case it had no effect.

Command hallucinations are fearsome and so are the disciplinary practices of some un-hallucinated fathers. In a case that illustrates how coprophagia can be an obsessive-compulsive phenomenon, a 13-year-old boy who five years earlier had been forced to eat faeces by his father as a punishment, developed a powerful, guilt-riddled urge to repeat the act when his mother died. As he moved into young adulthood he continued to feel a compulsion to eat faeces whenever he had done something wrong, finding that this action diminished his anxiety. His coprophagia escalated as an apparently self-punishing response even when he had no grounds for feeling guilt, until a behavioural treatment for OCD brought it to an end by reducing his anxiety and bolstering his resistance to his compulsion of choice (Zeitlin & Polivy, 1995). The same compulsive quality was found in a Belgian woman whose 'scrupulous cleanliness' led her to fear soiling even her toilet bowl, driving her to hide or eat her faeces in an effort not to dirty herself or her surroundings (Leroy, 1929). Similarly, an American soldier reportedly had a compulsive urge to eat his own faeces, requiring sedation when a ward attendant once flushed his toilet before he had a chance to raid it. He was otherwise noted to be orderly in manner and very neat in his outward appearance, but dirty beneath, rarely changing his underclothes (Kessler & Poucher, 1945).

One fascinating case of coprophagia has been reported in the clinical literature within the context of a sexual fetish. Although the activity may play a role in some paraphilias (formerly known as perversions), in the case of this middle-aged married policeman (Wise & Goldberg, 1995), who was depressed and alcoholic, it became part of a masturbation ritual. The behaviour disappeared when his depression and alcohol abuse were successfully treated with a combination of antidepressant medications and psychotherapy.

A final motive for eating excrement is to pretend to be psychiatrically unwell. People may malinger for a variety of reasons, such as crying for help or attempting to evade punishment, and to do so they need to simulate mental illness. Unfortunately many malingerers have such a limited understanding of mental illness that their simulations are implausible. A fine set of examples can be found in an epidemic of uncommon psychiatric symptoms reported by criminal defendants facing a third conviction under California's 'Three strikes and you're out' law, which mandated very long minimum sentences (Jaffe & Sharma, 1998). Several defendants told of seeing little green men and one ate his own faeces in dramatic fashion, having stockpiled them over a period of several days. Evidently some people think that bizarre hallucinations and revolting actions are the essence of madness, although in fact both phenomena are relatively rare. These examples illustrate a more general finding that malingerers tend to believe that people with mental illness are more deviant and freakish than they are in fact. The uncomfortable truth of the matter is that there is less difference between disorder and normality than people tend to think.

Conclusions

This catalogue of coprophagia shows just how complex one simple behaviour can be. Eating excrement can serve many functions, reveal many disorders and express many thoughts and wishes. It can be a compensation for lack of interpersonal connection, a regression to infantile modes of oral incorporation, a source of gustatory pleasure, a sign of disinhibition, an act of submission to powerful but imaginary figures, a form of penance, a desperate attempt to be clean, a sexual turn-on, or a symbol of madness. It paints from a rich emotional palette that includes not only disgust but also shame, fear, sadness, horror, anxiety, guilt and enjoyment. No behaviour has only one possible meaning, but coprophagia is surely one of the most versatile.

7
Toilet Graffiti

Writing is one of humanity's greatest inventions, so great that it cannot always be confined to paper and computer screens. People have been writing in public spaces and on other people's property for millennia. The inscriptions they leave are now widely known as graffiti, or literally 'little scratchings'. As a genre of writing, graffiti have been controversial, valued by some as a form of artistic expression and criticized by others as mere vandalism. They have been hung from the satin walls of fashionable galleries and scrubbed from the sides of urban buildings by rehabilitated practitioners.

Graffiti have not gone unnoticed by researchers. Scholars have been keen to record, describe and understand this form of everyday expression for the past century, and have drawn several basic distinctions. Most out-of-place inscriptions can be classified as tourist graffiti, inner-city graffiti or toilet graffiti (Anderson & Verplanck, 1983). Tourist graffiti are scratched on rocks, trees and monuments by passing visitors and consist mainly of names, dates and simple expressions of affection. Roman soldiers left them on the pyramids during their occupation of Egypt, and hundreds of Greek and Latin inscriptions of the form 'Kilroy was here' have been found on rocks at a popular resting spot beside an ancient trail in Palestine. Inner-city graffiti tend to be more elaborate, featuring names, images and statements of identity painted on city walls, often staking territorial claims.

Toilet graffiti – dubbed 'latrinalia' by one scholar – appear on bathroom walls. They are produced in a setting that is an unusual mixture of private and public. All graffiti-writing requires a certain amount of secrecy, and bathroom stalls are more private than the spaces where other forms of graffiti are produced, allowing wall-scribblers more time and leisure to compose their messages. The chances of being caught in the act of writing are minimal if the latch is correctly engaged. Public bathrooms are also in some sense more public than other shared spaces, offering graffiti-writers a confined and captive audience with whom to communicate. Private bathrooms do not offer the same opportunities for graffiti. The only recorded example is a woman who, urged by a therapist to shake up her marriage by doing something bizarre, wrote 'Save the Whales!' in lipstick on her bathroom mirror. Her husband appreciated the humour, but his mother and aunt, seeing it on an unexpected visit, did not (Watson et al., 1992).

Toilet graffiti are affected by their context in two other important ways: they appear in a place that is associated with taboo activities and that is usually segregated by gender. Scatological ideas and images are likely to be highly salient to people in bathrooms and so we should not be surprised that they are expressed on bathroom walls more than on city streets and tourist sites. Gender is also salient: men and women are reminded of the category to which they belong when they enter a public bathroom and they can be reasonably confident that what they write will not be read by the opposition. As a result, latrinalia might be expected to highlight differences between men's and women's preoccupations and ways of thinking, and to contain uncensored records of what they think of one another.

In this chapter we explore the many intriguing dimensions of latrinalia, focusing on the findings of a surprisingly large body of psychological research and theory on this apparently fringe topic. After discussing the history of latrinalia, we examine how it can be classified, looking over the typical themes it expresses and the varied forms that it takes. We then investigate the range of factors that influence how toilet graffiti are expressed, examining differences due to gender, age, history, culture and personality. Finally we turn to the many theories that psychologists have proposed for why people write latrinalia at all and why it tends to be expressed in the ways that it is.

History

Graffiti have a long and ignoble history that extends back at least as far as the ancient Greeks, who from the sixth century

BC inscribed buildings in the Athenian agora with names, casual portraits, alphabets and the occasional sexual insult (Lang, 1988). Inhabitants of Pompeii left a rich record of wall scratchings, many of them obscene, although there is little evidence that these were confined to privies. However, latrinalia was a feature of Roman life at least by the time of the writer Martial, who in about AD 101 scolded a fame-seeking fellow poet by suggesting that he would only be published on a toilet wall:

> If you aim at getting your name into verse, seek, I advise you, some sot of a poet from some dark den, who writes, with coarse charcoal and crumbling chalk, verses which people read as they ease themselves

Some of the finest evidence of vintage latrinalia can be found in compilations collected from public houses by Hurlo Thrumbo, an Englishman of the early eighteenth century. Many of the inscriptions collected in his book *The merry-thought: or, the glass-window and bog-house miscellany* (1731) were scratched on windows and drinking glasses, but some disgraced the walls of public toilets, or 'bog-houses'. Most of his examples were rendered in verse and most deal with elimination in a humorous fashion, often mixed with gentle social critique. Some pass comment on the writing of graffiti itself:

No hero looks so fierce in fight
As does the man who strains to shite

If smell of Turd makes wit to flow
Laud I what would eating of it do

Good Lord! Who could think
That such fine Folks should stink?
[in a 'person of quality's boghouse']

Well sung of Yore, a Bart of Wit;
That some Folks read, but all Folks shit
But now the Case is alter'd quite,
Since all who come to Boghouse write

Scholarship devoted to graffiti has a shorter history. Even so, folklorists of the early twentieth century began to write about them in the obscure Austrian journal *Anthropophyteia*, which closed down under obscenity-based legal threats in 1913 despite Sigmund Freud's expressions of support. Under such headings as 'pissoirinschriften' and 'skatologische inschriften', scholars scoured the historical record and contemporary lavatories for examples of latrinalia. Reiskel (1906), for example, presents examples in Latin, French and German that are sometimes crude and insulting and at other times witty, poetic and even philosophical:

> Shit hard, shit soft
> But in the name of God, shit in the pot
>
> Here falls in ruin
> All the masterpieces of cuisine
>
> Love is a devouring fire
> The desire to shit is even stronger
>
> In this solitary place
> Where one comes to shit
> The mouth must be quiet
> And the arse must speak

After the demise of *Anthropophyteia* the study of latrinalia languished, with the notable exception of a collection brought out by Allen Walker Read in 1935. This tireless American folklorist documented graffiti from the western USA but published them in Paris, knowing that they would draw obscenity charges at home (Read, 1935). Despite these barren years, toilet graffiti research would soon come out of the (water) closet again.

The content of latrinalia

Latrinalia scholarship underwent a renaissance in the 1960s, 1970s and 1980s, boosted by the growing academic interest in low and popular forms of culture and in types of scholarship seen as transgressive. Whereas folklore researchers and other humanists catalogued graffiti and interpreted their meanings, psychologists began to count them, submit them to statistical analysis and examine how they varied among different groups: men and women, adults and children, liberals and conservatives, Americans and others. The most elementary task for these researchers, armed with their stacks of index cards or megabytes of images collected from public facilities, is to develop a classification of what they have found.

The task of classifying toilet graffiti is far from simple, as they are enormously varied. One attempt (Anderson & Verplanck, 1983) derived 14 categories: politics, humour, simple replies, sex, race, general insults, music, religion, Greek (i.e., fraternities and sororities), drugs, sports, nuclear-environmental, philosophical and miscellaneous. Even with classifications such as these some graffiti slip between the cracks or cannot be readily sorted into a single category. One group of researchers noted the difficulty of coding 'Fuck LBJ': is it political, hostile or sexual? Despite these difficulties, certain themes recur frequently enough to deserve mention.

Sexual

A large proportion of the graffiti found in men's bathrooms consists of homosexual solicitations for 'tea-room trade' (Abel & Buckley, 1977). Many researchers have found high proportions of this type of graffiti, which commonly describe genital attributes, desired sexual activities and times and places when they might be enjoyed (Innala & Ernulf, 1992). However, other kinds of sexual inscriptions also appear, often advocating self-sufficiency or advertising heterosexual opportunities of an ancient kind that only inflation has altered:

> Sex is like bridge – if you have a good hand you don't need a partner
>
> (Bruner & Kelso, 1980)
>
> Marion $25
>
> (Los Angeles, 1965)
>
> I am yours for 2 coppers
>
> (Pompeii, 79)

Love and relationships

Many toilet graffiti have romantic rather than erotic content, often affirming close relationships in simple and conventional ways. Others express desires for love or problems in it, some seeming to cry out for guidance:

> Chucky and Debbie, '73, '74, . . . ?
>
> (Gonos et al., 1976)

> I love and am loved by 2 men. Sharing love is *great* But I just can't handle two. What should I do?
>
> (Bruner & Kelso, 1980)

Insults and hostility

Just as some graffiti express love and longing, some express the opposite. Insults and other derogatory comments may be personal or group-based, disparaging women, ethnic groups, belief systems, members of rival institutions, or sexual minorities:

> You are full of shit
>
> (Anderson & Verplanck, 1983)

> Screw homos
>
> (Stocker et al., 1972)

Political

Toilet graffiti frequently express political opinions and slogans, especially in the higher education settings where many studies have been conducted. Sometimes these take the form of short slogans but more extensive statements of dogma can also be found:

> Kennedy for President
>
> The multi-ethnic working class must unite to overcome the post-industrial capitalist forces
>
> (Bartholome & Snyder, 2004)

Humour

Political graffiti such as the above tend to be unfunny, but latrinalia is frequently amusing, or at least intended to be. Jokes are staples of toilet-wall scribblings and they often have sexual or scatological content, evoked, no doubt, by the vivid presence of excretion and unclothed nether regions in the bathroom setting. One-liners and wordplay predominate, but funny verses are also common:

> Don't look up here, the joke's between your legs
>
> (Anderson & Verplanck, 1983)

> Women should be obscene and not heard

> Those who write on shithouse walls
> Roll their shit in little balls
> Those who read those words of wit
> Eat the little balls of shit

Self-referential graffiti

A surprising quantity of toilet graffiti, like the previous classic example of scatological graffiti, refers to the act of writing and reading graffiti. Sitting on the toilet seems to instil a contemplative frame of mind in which people can reflect on graffiti and the writing of them:

> You all need a good swift KICK IN THE ASS for writing on these walls
>
> (Bartholome & Snyder, 2004)

Scatology

Many latrinalia, like the previous example, take their inspiration from the processes and products of elimination. Many of these have an earthily humorous intent:

> Here I sit all broken-hearted
> Tried to shit and only farted

> Flush twice, it's a long way to the White House
>
> (Gonos et al., 1976)

It should be obvious from this short catalogue that the contents and themes of toilet graffiti are highly diverse and impossible to capture in a few neat categories. Many graffiti make up combinations – scatological political insults, sexual humour, self-referential hostility – and in most studies a large number of graffiti remain unclassifiable, testaments to their writer's idiosyncrasy.

The form of latrinalia

Whatever their varied contents, latrinalia may take a variety of forms or genres. Sometimes it is pictorial rather than verbal, often involving obscene images of genitals and sexual couplings, as well as offensive symbols and fanciful sketches of human and animal bodies, and especially faces. One study found lips to be commonly drawn, but only in women's toilets (Kinsey et al., 1953). The same may go for love hearts and smiley faces (Green, 2003). Mixed pictorial and verbal forms also appear, such as a pseudoscientific grid, complete with column headings (1–2, 3–5, 6–10, 10–15 and 16+) placed under the statement 'How many wipes before you were clean?' (Whiting & Koller, 2007).

As we have seen, verbal latrinalia often takes the form of short verse or doggerel, often humorous and with sexual or scatological content. Another popular genre is the bastardized proverb, in which a familiar expression is altered for comic effect. Nierenberg (1994) has collected a large number of such proverbs in the USA and Germany. In Nierenberg's view, proverbs offer a perfect target for the playful, parodic and anti-authoritarian spirit of latrinalia. By deliberately tweaking earnest statements of social values they poke fun at conventions and norms:

> Never pull off tomorrow what you can pull off today
>
> Practice makes pervert
>
> Behind every great man there's an asshole

Another humorous genre is the sequence of parodic statements, such as adulterated movie or song titles that share the same basic verbal structure (Longenecker, 1977). Rich in wordplay and often quickly degenerating into obscenity, such chains of verbal invention can be long and creative:

> 1) John Wayne is a closet queen
> 2) Ellery Queen is a closet john
> 3) Queen Elizabeth is a water closet [and so on]
>
> (Longenecker, 1977, p. 363)

The chained quality of these parody sequences reminds us that many graffiti are not simple self-expressions but are attempts to communicate with others. They invite replies and commonly receive them. This has been amply demonstrated by studies that have attempted to influence the process of graffiti production. One pair of researchers taped posters to the inside doors of several bathroom stalls, half of which were adulterated with a graffito (Buser & Ferreira, 1980). The level of occupancy of the two sets of stalls was determined to be equivalent by the ingenious method of comparing toilet-paper usage. Stalls with marked posters received nine times as many inscriptions as those with unmarked posters, indicating that bathroom graffiti-writing often involves responding to or being otherwise inspired by a previous communication. The exchanges that result are sometimes hostile and challenging, and sometimes helpful and supportive. For example, some graffiti are confessional:

> I sometimes wonder what I see in him. He practically calls me ugly to my face AND then wants to give me a gift he originally bought for someone else. Guess that's the price I pay for giving him my virginity too quickly. Any advice girls?
>
> I think we had the same boyfriend! Seriously though, he's now (finally) my ex and life has never been better. Good luck.
>
> (Butler, 2006, p. 27)

Male examples of this advice-seeking genre are rarer and perhaps more direct, as in the example below:

> If I'm on a bus & a girl looks at you for the entire trip is she interested?
>
> She's begging for it
>
> (Butler, 2006, p. 43)

Influences on latrinalia

Up until now we have surveyed the wide field of toilet graffiti as if their features were universal. However, graffiti vary widely across different types of person, context, culture and time. If we want to know *who* produces what sort of latrinalia and *when*, we need to explore some of these influences.

Sex differences

By far the most extensively studied aspect of toilet graffiti are differences between men's and women's productions. This line of research was pioneered by Alfred Kinsey and colleagues, of Kinsey Report fame. Surveying the walls of more than three hundred public toilets, male and female, they found that men made more inscriptions and 86 per cent of these had erotic content compared to only 25 per cent of women's (Kinsey et al., 1953). Women's inscriptions, in turn, were much more likely than men's to relate to romantic love. Kinsey and colleagues suggested that women's lesser tendency to produce erotic graffiti was due to their greater regard for moral codes and social conventions, and by their fundamentally weaker tendency to be aroused by the making and viewing of erotic graffiti. This general view that women's latrinalia are a little bit of a disappointment was expressed best by Lomas (1973), who dismissed them as 'sparse and unimaginative' (p. 76).

The sparseness of women's latrinalia may be a myth. Although several studies support Kinsey's finding that women produce fewer toilet graffiti (Landy & Steele, 1967; Peretti et al., 1977), others have found greater quantities of graffiti in women's restrooms (Ahmed, 1981; Bartholome & Snyder, 2004; Bates & Martin, 1980; Farr & Gordon, 1975; Wales & Brewer, 1976). It appears that over the past half-century women have caught up with and maybe surpassed men in this traditionally male activity.

Turning from quantity to quality, however, there does seem to be some truth to Kinsey's observation that male restrooms tend to contain more sexual graffiti than women's, although exceptions have been found (Ahmed, 1981; Bartholome & Snyder, 2004). This is certainly true when it comes to homosexual solicitations, but it also holds for heterosexual images, jokes and comments. The typically greater forthrightness about sexual matters in men's latrinalia is nicely illustrated by two parallel graffiti collected in the men's and women's bathrooms of a restaurant in Rochester, New York. There are no prizes for guessing which is which:

> People who live in glass houses should fuck in the basement
>
> People who live in glass houses should get intimate in the basement
>
> (Bartholome & Snyder, 2004)

There are many other apparent differences in the themes of men's and women's latrinalia. Men's tends to be more hostile and derogatory, more likely to contain racist or sexist comments, more argumentative and competitive, more humorous, especially regarding elimination, more likely to contain scatological content and expletives, and more political. Women's tends to be more confessional, more friendly, more likely to express solidarity with other women, more socially acceptable and more romance-related (Arluke et al., 1987; Bruner & Kelso, 1980; Green, 2003; Loewenstine et al., 1982; Schreer & Strichartz, 1997; Wales & Brewer, 1976).

Women differ not only in the content of the latrinalia they produce, but also in the form or manner in which they produce it. Men's toilet graffiti are more likely to be images, primarily anatomical. Women's latrinalia more often involves replies to existing items than men's, who are more likely to write stand-alone items (Bates & Martin, 1980; Stocker et al., 1972). Women tend to engage in more exchanges in which advice is sought and given, and inputs are generally helpful and sisterly. Sisterhood has its limits, however:

> Keep him, Donna, you whore
>
> (Bartholome & Snyder, 2004)

Women may even have different understandings of what graffiti are and why people produce them. One female study participant had a highly distinctive understanding, defining graffiti as 'tiny Italian giraffes' (Bruner & Kelso, 1980). A study found that women are less likely than men to see latrinalia as something that emanates from frustration and hostility – one man saying in reference to it that 'Everyone needs exploding space' (Bruner & Kelso, 1980) – and more likely to see it as a forum for resolving personal problems. Women also tend to find graffiti less socially acceptable (McMenemy & Cornish, 1993). Even so, men and women are in agreement that people who write toilet graffiti are funny but immature (Loewenstine et al., 1982).

The most scientifically impressive study of gender differences in toilet graffiti was conducted in New Zealand by James Green (2003). Green made important advances by developing an explanation for why gender differences might be especially notable in toilets and by comparing latrinalia with graffiti collected in a different, control location. He observed that public toilets make gender highly salient: signs alert us that only one gender is permitted in the room, we only see people of one gender entering and exiting it, and the biological act of excretion reminds us of our own gender. We might be tempted to see the toilet cubicle as a place where each gender reveals its true nature on the walls, unconstrained by the presence of the other. In fact, Green argued, our anonymity and the salience of our gender in public bathrooms are likely to polarize our behaviour so that we exaggerate our femaleness or maleness. If that is the case, then latrinalia might differ from the sorts of graffiti that people leave in other, less gender-marked locations.

To examine this possibility Green collected 723 inscriptions from male and female bathrooms in a university library, as well as from nearby study booths. The male bathroom graffiti were distinctive in having the highest rate of racist comments, political content, insults, statements of presence ('I was here'), expletives and images. Female latrinalia contained more discussions of rape, religion, personal advice, body image and love or romance. Women's toilet graffiti also tended to be longer, more personally disclosing, more likely to be a reply to an earlier graffito and more empathic. Men and women were about equal in their references to sex but with somewhat different focus: men's graffiti consisted mainly of requests and women's mainly involved giving or seeking sexual advice.

Study booths were different again. They tended to contain relatively high rates of insults, humour and content related to drinking, drugs and philosophy. They contained relatively low rates of male-typical latrinalia topics, with the exception of insults, and relatively low rates of female-typical material as well, with the exception of religion. They were also relatively lacking in sexual content compared to both male and female latrinalia. However, they frequently contained sexist remarks, which were clearly attempts to provoke people in a mixed-gender environment. In short, Green's predictions were largely borne out. Stereotypically masculine elements are played up in men's latrinalia and stereotypically feminine elements are presented in exaggerated form in women's. In the neutral, unsegregated zone of the study booth these gendered forms are relatively infrequent and with some exceptions the graffiti addressed familiar themes of mixed-gender college life: humour, insults, the meaning of life and substance use.

All in all, there is little that comes out of latrinalia research that challenges well-worn gender stereotypes. Men's toilet graffiti tend to be more libidinal and aggressive, more insulting, more visual, more individualistic and competitive, and less interactive. Women's tend to be more conventional, more controlled and polite, more friendly and communicative, more wordy and literate, and more preoccupied with love and relationships.

Historical changes

There have been few studies of historical shifts in the content of graffiti and these tend to emphasize changes related to gender. The main emphasis of this work has been on whether the gender gaps identified in early work by Kinsey and colleagues in the 1950s have narrowed in more recent years, in parallel with other signs of progress towards gender equality. Some studies suggest that the gap has indeed narrowed. Ahmed (1981) found that women no longer wrote fewer toilet graffiti than men and Farr and Gordon (1975) observed that they were also becoming more sexual and erotic in content. In contrast, other work finds the gap widening, with men's graffiti becoming even more sexual over time while women's stay constant, a finding that the study's authors attribute to men's growing insecurity in the face of changing relations between the sexes and the challenge these pose to their traditional roles (Arluke et al., 1987). Women's latrinalia became more political in content over this period, suggesting that political frictions between men and women may have been more heated than in previous decades.

Although some forms of toilet graffiti have increased over time, others have declined. Stocker et al. (1972) observed a decline in graffiti involving homosexual solicitations and predicted that they would die out within the next decade as societal attitudes liberalized and solicitations no longer needed to be hidden away.

Differences in social position

If historical changes in the content of toilet graffiti reflect changes in social roles and beliefs we might expect that people who occupy different roles and have different beliefs at any single point in time might also produce different kinds of graffiti. Researchers have examined a variety of differences of this sort, including those associated with different kinds of institutions, different social classes, and different social attitudes and ideologies. Graffiti tended to be more hostile and less likely to contain homosexual content in trade-school toilets than those in tertiary institutions frequented more by middle-class students (Sechrest & Olson, 1971), and female latrinalia at universities with wealthier student bodies also tends to have more erotic content than in poorer institutions. Higher rates of racist latrinalia are found in racially integrated schools than in segregated schools, implying that these graffiti reflect and express tensions and conflicts in the institution beyond the toilet cubicle (Wales & Brewer, 1976).

Just as toilet graffiti reflect institutional tensions, they reflect the basic preoccupations of their visitors. Comparing toilets in different faculties of one university, researchers found that Arts toilets contained more artistic and political content as well as poetry than graffiti in Law and Computer Science toilets (Landy & Steele, 1967). In another, political and musical content was especially prevalent in Humanities bathrooms, racial and insulting content in a business school, and sexual content, for some reason, among architects (Anderson & Verplanck, 1983).

Cultural differences

Although studies of toilet graffiti have been conducted in many countries, few systematic cross-cultural comparisons have been attempted. The first, by Sechrest and Flores (1969), collected graffiti in Chicago and Manila bathrooms and found that sexual content was much less frequent in the Philippines, as was scatological and philosophical content (e.g., 'God is dead . . . but so is Nietzsche'). In particular, graffiti related to homosexuality – whether solicitations, drawings or homophobic remarks – were almost absent there. The authors speculated that this finding reflected not a greater sexual openness among the Americans but instead a higher degree of conflict over homosexuality, which finds hidden expression in bathroom scribblings.

Cultural variations in the degree of political emphasis in latrinalia have also attracted interest from researchers. One study compared

French- and English-Canadian high-school students in Ontario and found the former's graffiti to be more political, consistent with their minority status within their country and province (Ahmed, 1981). Political content also dominated all other themes in a study conducted in a Nigerian university (Nwoye, 1993), consistent with an earlier study by Olowu (1983) that compared graffiti in the bathrooms of two English and two Nigerian universities. Here the similarities were as evident as the differences: local politics, heterosexual content and humour predominated in both countries. Stark differences emerged as well. There was no homosexual content in the Nigerian bathrooms, compared to 15 per cent of all inscriptions in England, and there were no references to supernatural, superstitious and animistic content in England, although these made up 12 per cent of the Nigerian graffiti. Studies such as these demonstrate that toilet graffiti reflect distinctive cultural preoccupations.

The absence of homosexual graffiti in Nigeria, a country where homosexuality is strictly taboo, raises questions about Sechrest and Flores' interpretation that the same absence implied heightened tolerance of homosexuality in the Philippines. What to make of these questions is unclear. A lack of homosexual graffiti could mean different things: a lack of social repression of homosexuality or such a powerful repression that the taboo extends even into the privacy of toilet stalls and makes men wary of advertising there. The presence of homosexual latrinalia could be a symptom of societal tolerance or intolerance, and so could its absence.

Age differences

Surprisingly little has been written on the latrinalia of children and adolescents. Studies of American high-school bathrooms (Gonos et al., 1976; Wales & Brewer, 1976) found that it was largely romantic in nature and lacking significant amounts of racist or otherwise prejudiced content. Unusually, girls were much more productive than boys in this age group. Sexual and scatological content were present, especially among boys, but sexual insults and erotic humour were also present in a small but significant minority of graffiti written by girls, especially those from wealthier backgrounds. Similar patterns of female specialization in romance and male focus on sex and scatology have been observed in Canadian and Brazilian high schools (Ahmed, 1981; Otta et al., 1996) but with some specific patterns: more politics in Canada and more sport in Brazil. Overall, though, high-school latrinalia appears to be generally more innocent – less hostile and sexually explicit – than what is found in university restrooms, although sexual messages can sometimes be the source of high-school girls' sexual harassment complaints (Walsh et al., 2007).

Very little work has been done on the latrinalia of younger children, but two studies of elementary school students' wall scribblings shine a revealing light. Early adolescent latrinalia seems to revolve around themes of sexual maturity, identity, idealism and iconoclasm and rebelliousness (Peretti et al., 1977). Boys' scratchings tend to be more preoccupied with sexual knowingness ('James fucked Shirley') and attacks on belief systems ('Religion is shit'), whereas girls' contains more self-evaluations ('I like guys who are honest') and visions of the future ('Things will be better when I grow up'). Both girls and boys revealed concerns with the onrush of adult sexuality and the leaving behind of childish illusion and dependency.

Even younger children also leave graffiti that express their developmental stage. A study of 6- to 11-year-olds in Puerto Rico (Lucca & Pacheco, 1986) found that the children's toilet graffiti were dominated by romantic statements, obscenities and especially autographs, suggesting that graffiti express personal identity among children even more than among adolescents. Humour, religion and politics were largely absent, but drawings were also much more common than in studies of adults. Boys tended to draw genitalia whereas girls tended to leave simple scratch-marks and stick figures, using rude and dirty words more than images of the things they signify. Both boys and girls frequently wrote insults and verbal attacks; most often, for girls, against their female peers. The frequency with which romantic sentiments were expressed suggested that even at age 6 the children had a sense of sex-roles and sex differences.

Personality differences

The personality of the bathroom graffitist has received little scientific attention, for the obvious reason that it is difficult to catch scribblers in the act and persuade them to complete a questionnaire. Several distinct personality profiles could be anticipated depending on one's beliefs about the nature of the scribbler's motivations. If bathroom graffiti are the product of sexual frustration we might expect their creators to be immature and impulsive. If it is a way of thumbing one's nose at authority, they might be antisocial, rebellious and aggressive. If it is a way of expressing sentiments that the person cannot express in public, they might be shy and introverted. The complete personality profile of the bathroom graffiti-writer has yet to be determined, but two studies have made a start.

Schwartz and Dovidio (1984) asked college students how they indulged in private graffiti – on walls or desks – and compared those who never wrote and those who did at least sometimes. The writers scored higher on a test of creativity than the non-writers, tended to believe that their destiny and the consequences of their behaviour were less under their personal control and, not surprisingly, felt more favourably towards graffiti. The researchers concluded that graffiti are more a purposeful expression of personal creativity than a form of destructiveness, although on one reading of their findings the graffiti-writers were simply less conventional and more alienated than their non-scrawling peers.

Different conclusions follow from a study that compared the authoritarian tendencies of frequent and infrequent toilet graffiti-writers (Solomon & Yager, 1975). If graffiti-writing simply represented a benign flowering of creativity then anti-authoritarians would tend to do more of it, but the opposite pattern was observed. Frequent writers scored higher on a survey assessing conformity, submission to traditional authority and punitiveness towards people who violate social norms. In this study much of the graffiti that were observed were anti-gay and hostile to members of other groups, a kind of latrinalia for which authoritarians might have special gifts. There may be no single kind of personality associated with writing on toilet walls. Instead, different personalities may be implicated depending on the tone and content of the graffiti. Creativity may underpin some kinds of writing and intolerant social ideologies may underpin others. The definitive study remains to be done.

Theories of latrinalia

As we have seen, toilet graffiti are diverse and influenced by many factors. We know a good deal about what they are like and what shapes them, but why do people produce them in the first place? Explaining latrinalia – what drives people to scribble on toilet walls and why they give it the forms they do – is a different and more challenging matter, but theorists have put forward a variety of explanations. Some emphasize psychological factors in their explanations whereas others place societal factors in the foreground. Similarly, some theorists see toilet graffiti as a relatively straightforward reflection of individual minds or social values, whereas others see the determining factors as hidden forces. Put these two dichotomies together and we have four kinds of theory: latrinalia is understood as a simple reflection of people's everyday thoughts and desires, as a product of hidden psychological dynamics, as a reflection of dominant social values, or as a symptom of underlying societal conflicts.

Latrinalia as a reflection of individual psychology

Perhaps the simplest and most commonsense explanation of toilet graffiti is that they merely reveal well-known facts about human psychology. By this kind of account, the content and form of latrinalia are a direct manifestation of our attitudes, values and motives. Kinsey and colleagues (1953), for example, interpreted the paucity and undersexed nature of women's graffiti as further evidence of their weaker erotic responsiveness to visual stimuli and their greater social propriety compared to men. In the same manner, other researchers have read gender differences in the content of latrinalia as a straightforward manifestation or 'nonreactive measure' of gender differences in attitudes (Bates & Martin, 1980). If men and women produce different kinds of toilet graffiti, these differences are presumed to correspond to basic differences in male and female personality and sexuality. On this view, latrinalia merely reinforces what we think we already know about gender and tends to confirm our stereotypes. As Green's (2003) work shows, however, the picture of gender that appears on restroom walls may be deceptive: men and women may be exaggerating their stereotypic masculinity and femininity because the bathroom makes this distinction so vividly present to them.

Latrinalia as a product of hidden psychodynamics

Several writers have approached latrinalia as a less direct but no less meaningful manifestation to human psychology. Instead of seeing it simply as a mirror of our attitudes and personalities, these psychoanalytic writers view toilet graffiti as a 'self-administered projective test of individuals and society' (Gadpaille, 1974, p. 73) and as a safety-valve for taboo ideas and wishes. In principle, latrinalia could be interpreted as eruptions of Unconscious desires just as much as a person's responses to inkblots, or their dreams and slips of the tongue. The key proposition of this kind of explanation is that people may not be aware of what drives them to scribble on bathroom walls and that their scribblings cannot be taken at face value.

These psychoanalytic readings of toilet graffiti have been very diverse. One of the simplest argues that graffiti-writing is a form of 'phallic expression' and hence something more in men's natures than women's. Noting that male toilet stalls tended to be generally filthier than female stalls and more covered in graffiti, but that female stalls contained more cigarette butts, early theorists (Landy & Steele, 1967) speculated that whereas men's phallic needs are discharged by wielding pens on walls, women's is discharged by smoking: 'males act out this need by creating graffiti, females smoke it out!' (p. 712). Although Kinsey interpreted the apparent sex differences in graffiti as mere reflections of male and female psychology, he also engaged in some speculations on their unconscious meanings, musing that many depictions of male anatomy and sexual function were made by ostensibly heterosexual men who had unconscious homosexual wishes.

These writers see the psychodynamics of toilet graffiti primarily in terms of sexuality, but other psychoanalytic explanations have looked elsewhere. Gadpaille (1974) sees toilet graffiti-writing as a form of aggression, in which scribblers defy social prohibitions by mocking and violating cultural taboos. Aggression is also the main motif in the analysis of Harvey Lomas (1973, 1976, 1980), who interprets toilet graffiti as hostile attacks on the restroom wall itself. Walls represent our separation from one another and remind us of our isolation. Toilet graffiti are therefore a form of aggressive protest against the wall for what it represents and a kind of exhibitionistic hostility towards the captive audience that is forced to view it. The restroom wall is also a blank screen onto which our unsatisfied desires can be projected, and, in the graphic scribblings he witnesses, Lomas sees evidence of the persistence in adulthood of the infant's 'polymorphously perverse' sexuality.

The most intriguing psychoanalytic explanation of latrinalia comes from Alan Dundes (1966), who coined the term. In what he called an exercise in 'hard core ethnography', Dundes suggests that there is a distinctly anal erotic aspect to latrinalia and that it is akin to faecal smearing. Dirty words on bathroom walls are symbolically equivalent to excrement and by writing them people are releasing the childish impulses towards bodily filth that are normally sublimated in adulthood. Dundes goes further and suggests that this anal dynamic may help to explain men's greater propensity to write latrinalia. Men unconsciously envy women their capacity for childbirth and see defecation as an alternative. Women, needing no such alternative, are less in need of 'faecal substitute activities' such as latrinalia, painting, sculpture and the playing of wind instruments. For all its far-fetchedness and its inability to account for women's substantial graffiti production, Dundes' account does find at least some resonance in one of the ancient boghouse graffiti collected by Thrumbo in the early eighteenth century:

> Hard stools proceed from costive Claret
> Yet mortal Man cannot forbear it
> So Child-bed Women, full of Pain
> Will grunt and groan, and to't again

Latrinalia as a reflection of dominant social values

If we turn to accounts of toilet graffiti that emphasize social factors rather than psychological dynamics, we find some that read a culture or group's values or concerns directly off the prevalence of certain kinds of graffiti in their public restrooms. The greater prevalence of homosexual graffiti in the USA than in the Philippines (Sechrest & Flores, 1969) has been taken as evidence of more tolerant social attitudes in the latter. Similarly, the lessening of homosexual solicitations in toilet graffiti has been interpreted as a straightforward outcome of liberalizing social attitudes (Stocker et al., 1972). In the same fashion, findings that poetry, art and politics are more common in the graffiti of humanities students (Landy & Steele, 1967) and that supernatural content is more common in Nigerian latrinalia than British (Olowu, 1983), can be viewed as relatively self-evident parallels between the cultural preoccupations of a group and the themes of its wall scratching. All of these examples represent commonsense ways in which writers have understood toilet graffiti as social attitudes and values writ small.

Latrinalia as a societal symptom

Other writers have been at pains to challenge this way of reading social attitudes off bathroom walls. Toilet graffiti may refract rather than reflect society. Some writers have gone so far as to propose that graffiti may be inversely related to a society's dominant values. On this view, when some values become dominant it leads people to express their opposition to these values in covert and underground ways, such as by scrawling anonymously in a bathroom stall. Thus, homophobic graffiti may increase as social attitudes become less anti-gay and racist graffiti may be more prevalent in liberal academic settings, where expression of racist sentiments is less acceptable, than in other public settings (Gonos et al., 1976). Likewise, nastier forms of graffiti may appear in times and places where positive social change is underway, but where conflicts and suppressed resentments of those who feel threatened and left behind by history find their way onto restroom walls. This kind of social dynamic presumably accounts for the much higher frequency of racist graffiti in integrated schools than in those that are racially segregated (Wales & Brewer, 1976). In each of these cases, toilet graffiti do not merely reflect dominant values, but react and rebel against them as the symptomatic expression of hidden conflict and dissent.

Hidden social dynamics of another sort have also been proposed in analyses of gender differences in graffiti. Bruner and Kelso (1980) argue that beneath the surface of these differences – men's typically more sexual, aggressive, derogatory and competitive themes, women's more interactive and advisory style – lie differences in power. Men's graffiti, they argue, signify male dominance and are written by men to remind themselves and one another of their superiority and control. Women's graffiti signify the 'cooperation of the dominated' and the tendency both to muse on the nature of their subordination to men and to help one another deal with or resist that predicament. In short, a hidden political dynamic lurks behind bathroom wall-writing.

It need hardly be said that no explanation of latrinalia can be complete and each one, if it has any merit at all, is partial. Some explanations have more to say about men's typically more erotic and hostile graffiti than women's. Some fare best as attempts to make sense of gender differences, others as efforts to account for expressions of social prejudice. Together they show that toilet graffiti can bring to light our preoccupations and desires, both superficial and hidden, as well as revealing the norms and the taboos of our cultures and social environments. What they all do is remind us of the richness and complexity of latrinalia and our inability to understand it with unaided common sense. Toilet graffiti may be scribbled in moments of bored solitude, but they also have a lot to tell us about the mind and society.

Conclusions

As we have seen, latrinalia opens a revealing window on gender, psychological development, sexuality, culture and the rich diversity of people's hidden thoughts. There is something about the location of this form of half-forbidden writing that makes it so revealing. The public toilet is a space that is private but shared, anonymous but intimate, and linked in the mind to our bodies, our genders and sexuality. Even so, toilet graffiti seem to have fallen off the cultural radar in recent times. Research devoted to them has slowed since the glory years of the 1970s and 1980s and they are no longer the focus of the same amount of everyday interest. What gives?

One possibility is that they have gone digital. Why scribble scurrilous comments on bathroom walls for a meagre one-at-a-time audience when you can make the same remarks on a discussion board or chatroom to a large and simultaneous readership? Why solicit sexual partners with a crude drawing when websites can direct you to people who are more likely to be receptive to it than a random bathroom visitor seeking relief of a different sort? Online communication can offer the same kind of anonymity, privacy and freedom from restraint as the toilet cubicle, but in turbo-charged form. We should hardly be surprised that it often contains the same kinds of offensiveness, insult, prejudice, playfulness and sexual and aggressive content as toilet graffiti, its rather quaint precursor.

8
Seat Up or Down?

The bathroom is one of the key battlefields in the gender wars. Skirmishes may erupt over toothpaste-tube etiquette, soap fragrances, towel placement and general cleanliness, but the most enduring and heated conflict tends to focus on the toilet seat. In mixed-sex households disagreements often arise over whether the seat should always be left in the down position. Often the woman is angered that the man leaves the seat up after doing his business and sees this as evidence of selfishness, insensitivity and even sexism. Often the man cannot see what all the fuss is about, or why he should drop the seat for her if she does not raise it for him.

As conflicts between the sexes go, this one seems rather trivial and absurd. In one respect it involves moving a light object a small distance. In another respect it is quite basic. More than most other conflicts it derives fairly directly from the anatomical difference between the sexes: it is convenient for him to stand while urinating but not for her. Freud argued that the psychology of gender ultimately derives from this difference – that anatomy is destiny – but usually its link to gender differences in behaviour, taste and attitude is obscure or non-existent. But in this case, at least, the answer to Freud's eternal question – 'What do women want?' – is very clear. Put the seat down!

The psychology of toilet-seat behaviour turns out to be unexpectedly complex and revealing. In this chapter I develop an empirically based analysis of the rhythm of toilet use in an average mixed-sex bathroom and take it as a basis for investigating four alternative ways in which men and women might deal with the toilet-seat issue.

From this analysis I determine which strategy is the most rational, efficient and fair. The limitations of this analysis lead to an investigation of why an inquiry into this matter cannot be resolved in quasi-economic terms and why, instead, we need to consider psychological factors. The emotional resonance of the toilet-seat issue demands an analysis that goes beyond issues of efficiency and rationality narrowly conceived, and brings to the surface matters to do with basic human motives and desires.

Toilet-seat behaviour

To understand the rationality or otherwise of different toilet-seat regimes we first need an analysis of people's toileting habits. How often are men and women who share a toilet likely to avail themselves of it and how often are they likely to encounter its seat in particular configurations? Let's imagine the situation of an average heterosexual couple, Jack and Jill.

There is plenty of good excretory science on which to estimate our couple's toileting patterns. A survey of British adults, funded in part by the Kellogg Company, ascertained that the most common 'interdefecatory interval' for both men and women was about 24 hours and the most common weekly defecation frequency was seven (Heaton et al., 1992). Although daily regularity is the most common pattern, more than 60 per cent of adults departed from it. But let our generic Jack and Jill be blessedly regular.

Number ones tend to be more common than number twos. Surveys of adults indicate that men between the ages of 20 and 70 tend to urinate seven times in a 24-hour period (rising from about six in their twenties to about eight in their sixties), whereas women's average is about eight (van Haarst et al., 2004). If we make the reasonable assumption that one of these urinations occurs during a defecation episode, Jack can be expected to visit the toilet seven times (six times for number 1 only) and Jill eight times. Nine of the 15 daily toilet visits will take place in a seated position.

The rhythm of toileting

We are now in a position to describe systematically the rhythm of toileting in a mixed-sex household: who does what and who follows.

Jack and Jill are unlikely to intersperse their toilet activities in a completely random sequence, nor are they likely to follow a strict alternating pattern. Jack and Jill will usually follow one another given the natural spacing of bowel and bladder voiding, but both will sometimes use the toilet twice in a row. Jill will also visit the bathroom slightly more often than Jack. So let's work out probabilities of different sequences of consecutive toilet episodes.

Let's start with Jack's urination-onlys, which we'll call $Jack_1$s. If Jack and Jill's toilet visits were randomly spaced there would be a 53 per cent chance of Jill using the toilet next and a 47 per cent chance of Jack (she goes eight times to his seven). Let's assume that having voided he's less likely to return in the near future. On this basis let's approximately halve his likelihood of being next to 20 per cent so that Jill's probability of being next is 80 per cent. If Jack defecates ($Jack_2$) on every seventh toilet visit, then the likelihood of a $Jack_2$ occurring after a $Jack_1$ is about one in six. So of the 20 per cent of occasions when Jack is the first person to use the toilet after one of his $Jack_1$s, about 3 per cent will be for $Jack_2$ and 17 per cent will be for another $Jack_1$.

What happens after $Jack_2$s? Again, let's say the likelihood of Jill paying the next visit is 80 per cent given that Jack is temporarily relieved of his burden. Jack is now highly unlikely to pay an immediate second visit for a $Jack_2$. In the absence of dodgy seafood these will rarely occur in quick succession, so let's downgrade the likelihood of one $Jack_2$ immediately following another to 2 per cent. The remaining option ($Jack_2$-$Jack_1$) takes up the remaining 18 per cent.

When Jill uses the toilet, she would have a 53 per cent likelihood of being the next user if our couple's toilet visits were distributed randomly. If we again approximately halve this likelihood to account for her temporary relief, the probability that Jill will succeed herself to the throne will be 30 per cent. Therefore Jack is likely to be the next user 70 per cent of the time. $Jack_1$s should be six times more probable than $Jack_2$s, so there is a 60 per cent chance that Jill's toilet use will be followed by a $Jack_1$ and 10 per cent by a $Jack_2$. Table 8.1 summarizes these calculations.

We now have a principled way of estimating what will transpire during an average day in Jack and Jill's bathroom. Table 8.2 presents the expected frequencies of each of the nine possible sequences of toilet use in an average day, based on the frequency of each use type by Jack and Jill and the probabilities that each particular use type

Table 8.1 Probability of second toilet-use types depending on first use type

First use type	Second use type		
	Pr($Jack_1$)	Pr($Jack_2$)	Pr(Jill)
$Jack_1$	0.17	0.03	0.80
$Jack_2$	0.18	0.02	0.80
Jill	0.60	0.10	0.30

Table 8.2 Expected frequencies of different toilet-use sequences in an average day

Use sequence	Frequency of first use	Conditional probability of second use	Expected frequency of sequence
$Jack_1$-$Jack_1$	6	0.17	1.02
$Jack_1$-$Jack_2$	6	0.03	0.18
$Jack_1$-Jill	6	0.80	4.80
$Jack_2$-$Jack_1$	1	0.18	0.18
$Jack_2$-$Jack_2$	1	0.02	0.02
$Jack_2$-Jill	1	0.80	0.80
Jill-$Jack_1$	8	0.60	4.80
Jill-$Jack_2$	8	0.10	0.80
Jill-Jill	8	0.30	2.40

will follow. As we can see, the most common sequences are Jill followed by $Jack_1$ and $Jack_1$ followed by Jill. These 9.6 gender-alternating sequences, in which the toilet-seat configuration has to change, are where the trouble all starts.

Strategies of toilet-seat positioning

Knowing the expected sequences of toilet use and their relative frequency we are now in a position to test several alternative ways in which the disposition of the toilet seat could be organized. Let me describe four possible strategies, the relative merits of which will be examined later. The implications of each strategy for the raising and lowering of the seat, for each of the nine toilet-use sequences, are presented in Table 8.3. These implications are confined to the first toilet user's seat movements after use and the second user's seat movements prior to use.

Table 8.3 Implications of the four strategies for each toilet-use sequence (seat movements required after 1st use and before 2nd use)

Use sequence	Self-reliance	Golden rule	Female-favouring	Male-favouring
$Jack_1$-$Jack_1$		⬇⬆	⬇⬆	
$Jack_1$-$Jack_2$	⬇	⬇	⬇	⬇
$Jack_1$-Jill	↓	⬇	⬇	↓
$Jack_2$-$Jack_1$	⬆	⬆	⬆	⬆
$Jack_2$-$Jack_2$				⬆⬇
$Jack_2$-Jill				⬆↓
Jill-$Jack_1$	⬆	↑	⬆	↑
Jill-$Jack_2$		↑⬇		↑⬇
Jill-Jill		↑↓		↑↓
Jack's moves	5.16	8	12	2
Jill's moves	4.8	10.4	0	16
Total moves	9.96	18.4	12	18

Note: ↑ Jill lifts, ↓ Jill drops, ⬆ Jack lifts, ⬇ Jack drops

a) *Self-reliance*. The simplest strategy toilet users might take is to place the seat in the position they need and leave it there when they are finished. In short, this is a strategy of present-focused self-reliance, with no thought for who will next use the toilet. In five of our nine toilet-use sequences the second user finds the seat in the desired position and no action is necessary. However, after $Jack_1$s Jill will need to drop the seat, as will Jack if a $Jack_2$ comes next. Similarly, Jack will need to lift the seat if Jill or $Jack_2$ precedes his intended $Jack_1$.

b) *Golden rule*. A second strategy involves showing consideration for the next user by anticipating the seat position that he or she will desire. It follows the 'golden rule' of doing unto others as one would have them do unto oneself. After each use of the toilet the person guesses who is likely to use the toilet next and adjusts the seat position as appropriate. As Table 8.1 shows, the most likely user after Jack is Jill and the most likely user after Jill is Jack, who will tend to be planning a $Jack_1$. Thus, Jack should drop the seat after $Jack_1$s and leave it down after $Jack_2$s. Jill should raise the seat when she is done. This strategy will sometimes generate double-movements of the seat.

After urinating Jack will drop the seat but then have to raise it again if the next toilet use is another $Jack_1$. Similarly, Jill will raise the seat after using it but if the following toilet use is hers or a $Jack_2$ then the seat will need to be re-lowered.

c) *Female-favouring.* A third strategy involves taking the seat-down position as the default and requiring the person who lifts the seat to immediately restore it to its rightful position. After urinating, Jack will drop the seat and have to lift it again if a $Jack_1$ is the next toilet use. If a Jill or $Jack_2$ precedes a $Jack_1$ he will have to lift the seat. This strategy is female-favouring because all seat movements are carried out by Jack.

d) *Male-favouring.* Our fourth strategy is the mirror image of the third as it systematically advantages the male by taking his favoured seat-up position as the default. Jill must lift the seat after each use, as must Jack after his $Jack_2$s. Jack will have to drop the already lifted seat when he prepares for a $Jack_2$ and Jill will have to do the same. Double-movements – lift then drop – will be required whenever two $Jack_2$s or Jills occur consecutively, or when one is followed by the other.

Evaluating the strategies

So how do our four strategies compare and which is the most sensible to adopt? This not a straightforward question, as there are at least two criteria we might use to answer it. The most sensible strategy might be the one that is the most efficient, in the sense of requiring the fewest overall seat movements. These movements take effort, and contact with the seat may be mildly aversive to some people, so minimizing movements is a worthy goal. Alternatively, the most sensible strategy might be the one that is the most fair and equitable. Any strategy that places a disproportionate burden on Jack or Jill might be undesirable, regardless of its efficiency. If Jack and Jill are a modern couple, it is likely that they would endorse fairness and equality as guiding principles of their relationship.

The top of Table 8.3 tells us how many seat movements Jack and Jill make in each toilet-use sequence for each of the four strategies. If we combine this information with the expected frequency of each sequence, shown in Table 8.2, then we discover how many seat movements Jack and Jill are likely to make during the average day. The last three rows of Table 8.3 present these estimates for each strategy: Jack's moves, Jill's moves and their combined total. The most efficient strategy is the one with the fewest total movements and the most equitable is the one in which Jack's and Jill's movements are most equal.

It is plain to see that the *Self-reliance* strategy is the most efficient. It requires only about ten seat movements in the average day (i.e., 2/3 of the time the toilet is used). The *Female-favouring* (seat-down default) strategy is only slightly less efficient. The least efficient are the *Golden rule* and *Male-favouring* strategies, both of which require almost twice as many seat movements as *Self-reliance*. These inefficient strategies both require frequent double-movements in which a first user's considerate anticipation of the next user's needs turns out to be inaccurate (*Golden rule*) or a rule-governed return to the seat-up default position by a first user must be reversed when the second user must also be seated (*Male-favouring*). The key advantage of the *Self-reliance* strategy is that unlike all other strategies it requires no seat movements to be made after the toilet has been used. All movements are made by the person who needs them at the time of their need.

But what about fairness? Is *Self-reliance* the most efficient but the least equitable, like turbo-capitalism? On the contrary, it is the most equitable of all, requiring Jack to make only slightly more toilet-seat movements than Jill. The *Golden rule* strategy is also quite equitable, requiring somewhat more work from women. The *Female-favouring* and *Male-favouring* strategies are, of course, the least equitable. The former allows Jill's hands to remain entirely unacquainted with the toilet seat. The latter requires Jack to sully himself only on the rare occasions when, in preparation for a $Jack_2$, he must drop the seat that had been raised for his benefit and when, in its aftermath, he must raise the seat in anticipation of a future $Jack_1$.

In sum, *Self-reliance* emerges as a rather unlikely winner among our four strategies, the most efficient and the most equitable of them all. The *Golden rule* and *Female-favouring* strategies compete for second place, the former equitable but highly inefficient and the latter efficient but highly inequitable. The *Male-favouring* strategy clearly comes last.

Is that all there is?

This analysis indicates that *Self-reliance* is clearly the best way to conduct toilet etiquette in mixed-sex households. Attending myopically and selfishly to the immediate demands of one's own excretion is not only the most efficient approach – the least soiling of hands and taxing of toilet-seat hinges – but it also comes closest to gender equity. Being considerate by anticipating the seat-positioning needs of the next user, including one's future self in Jack's case, is markedly inefficient and less equitable, with the burden falling on women more than men. Strategies that impose default seat positions are less efficient than *Self-reliance* and dispense with any semblance of gender-neutrality.

Will people now cheerfully accept the wisdom of self-reliance where toilet-seat etiquette is concerned? My strong suspicion is that most will not. Many men will feel vindicated in 'doing what comes naturally'. Many women will feel that this is not an issue to be resolved by a quasi-economic analysis and that what is at stake is men doing what is right – what *should* be done – rather than what is rational, fair or equitable in some abstract or mathematical sense. Indeed, women tend to be less predisposed to economic thinking (Bansak & Starr, 2010) and less prone to reason about human affairs in terms of costs, benefits, utilities and optimization, perhaps a key reason why economics is by far the most male-dominated of the social sciences. For women who are bothered by the toilet-seat question and of course for many happily domesticated men as well, the issue is moral and qualitative – whether a rule of good bathroom conduct is obeyed or broken – not prudent and quantitative.

This really does seem to be the nub of the issue. The disposition of toilet seats is often seen in moral terms. The emotions generated by incorrect dispositions are moral emotions: the righteous anger of the accuser and the righteous indignation of the wrongly (he thinks) accused. The responses to failures to lower the seat – anecdotally ranging from harsh words to sex-strikes to poisoning fantasies– are clearly moral punishments. The clue that moral considerations swirl around the toilet seat is the apparent triviality of the transgression and the seriousness with which it is assessed. Indeed, it is the triviality of the required action – a gravity-assisted post-flush nudge by the man's index finger – that contributes to the perceived seriousness of the transgression.

If the disposition of the toilet seat is a moral issue, in what way is this so? Many moral issues implicate harm and rights, but it is questionable whether these are involved here. There is no obvious right to have a toilet seat placed in a personally convenient position. There is also no obvious physical harm involved. What harm is being done to Jill when Jack leaves the toilet seat in the upward position in which he used it rather than lowering it in anticipation of her preference? Remember that there is a substantial likelihood that he will be the next toilet user and that he will again want the seat up if he is. The harm seems minimal. Jill incurs no pain or significant muscular or cognitive effort if she has to lower the seat. Having to touch the seat may induce some feelings of aversion, but if this is the case then protecting Jill from emotional harm by lowering the seat will inflict the same harm on Jack (i.e., robbing Peter to pay Pauline).

Seat positioning as a moral issue

So why does so much emotional heat and moral censure attach to the matter of the toilet seat? Or alternatively, what crucial additional factor does our analysis of the rhythms of toileting omit? Let's consider a few options:

1) *The trauma theory*. Anecdotal reports and cartoons tell of women who, making a nocturnal visit to the toilet, fall in because the previous user failed to lower the seat. Failure to protect the women by leaving this dangerous diameter would indeed be a matter of immoral carelessness. However, this possibility seems like a weak basis for imposing a seat-down prescription because it is likely to be rare and unlikely to be repeated and it does not seem entirely reasonable to hold Jack responsible for Jill's failure to check the seat's position. It is also possible for Jack to be the victim of his own failure to put the seat down, but men rarely if ever express fears of falling in or see the possibility as a reason to change their habit of leaving the seat up. In short, the trauma theory seems to be an attempt to rationalize a seat-down preference that has a less rational basis.

2) *The default position theory*. People tend to judge negatively actions that depart from a norm and believe that what is normal is also morally correct. The seat-down position is in some sense the norm, as it applies for 60 per cent of all toilet episodes in our hypothetical household. It is absolutely the norm for Jill, who never uses the seat-up position (except for a possible non-traditional toilet use), so she is likely to see the down position as the one where the seat 'belongs'. For Jack, of course, the seat-up position is the norm,

because he only puts the seat down for a minority of his toilet uses. This leaves a situation where Jack and Jill have different senses of what the norm is and thus a tendency to moralize departures from that norm. Jill has overall descriptive truth on her side, but also perhaps a greater tendency to see her non-preferred seat position as a deviation from the default position.

3) *The aesthetic preference theory*. Some women justify their preference for the seat-down position on aesthetic grounds: the seat simply looks better or more natural in that position. By leaving the seat up men are violating rules of good taste and therefore to be condemned. The grounds for this aesthetic preference are unclear, but may be supported by an unconscious recognition that the down position is more in accordance with gravity.

4) *The household labour theory*. A third account of the moral offence caused by men's leaving the seat up is that women still tend to do the bulk of the cleaning in most households. One study found that cleaning the toilet was seen as the third-most female-dominated household task out of 25 (Beckwith, 1992), at least in part because it shares many of the features that distinguish women's domestic tasks from men's: low status, frequent, not discretionary and indoors (Coltrane, 1989). If his urinary splatter becomes her sanitary problem then she has a legitimate hygienic grievance. It's a moral grievance too, because the splatter is under Jack's voluntary control, easily avoided by sitting down.

5) *The chivalric residue theory*. Another explanation, popular with some men, is that some women expect men to look after and protect them in a way that is not reciprocal. Just as Sir Walter Raleigh is said to have laid his cloak on a mud-puddle so that Queen Elizabeth I could walk over it without sullying her regal shoes, Jack should follow the *Female-favouring* strategy to protect Jill from the cloacal dirt of the toilet. According to this view, Jill takes Jack's failure to put the seat down as evidence of a lack of proper manly concern. A possible error of omission has become a definite sin of commission. Jill feels no obligation to show similar concern for Jack by lifting the seat to protect his finer feelings.

6) *The sexism theory*. One view of the toilet-seat issue is that leaving the seat up involves an in-your-face display of male privilege, a blatant insistence on male difference. According to this position, men should leave the seat down to express their equality with women,

making it an anti-sexist gesture, although it must be remembered that equality in seat placement means inequality in toilet-seat movements (i.e., the *Female-favouring* strategy). This view of gender toilet equality seems to underpin the development of a social norm of men sitting to urinate in Germany, where foreign visitors who leave the seat up are zealously corrected. The sexism theory does seem to have a measure of psychological reality, as some men do take standing urination as a valued male prerogative and disparage perceived femininity in other men by stating that they must sit (or squat) to pee.

7) *The disgust theory.* When Jack leaves the seat up, Jill often has to put it down. Touching the toilet evokes disgust for many people and is aversive for that reason. There is ample evidence that women tend to be more disgust-sensitive than men, including in the 'core disgust' domain of excretion (Haidt et al., 1994). One study found that fewer than 10 per cent of men were more disgust-prone than the average woman (Druschel & Sherman, 1999) and another found that women had much more negative attitudes to bodily elimination products (Templer et al., 1984). Women are therefore likely to have stronger aversions than men to anything connected with toilets, including touching their seats, and more likely to fear contamination by them. Our analysis of different strategies for toilet-seat placement, which proclaimed *Self-reliance* as the most efficient and equitable, assumed that each movement of the seat was equally unpleasant and effortful for Jack and Jill and aimed to minimize seat-touches. But what if moving the seat is more unpleasant on average for Jill? The analysis presented earlier implies that if each touch of the toilet seat is somewhat more aversive to Jill than Jack – at least 43 per cent to be precise – then the *Female-favouring* strategy is better than *Self-reliance* in minimizing the overall aversiveness of toilet-seat movement. Assuming a modestly greater female predisposition to find toilet-seat touching to be disgusting, a simple utilitarian analysis therefore suggests that men should put the seat down.

Conclusions

The definitive studies have yet to be conducted, but my guess is that the household labour, perceived sexism and disgust theories are the best accounts of why moral offence attaches to toilet-seat behaviour. They explain why leaving the seat up can be seen as immoral in three ways: because it inflicts undeserved harm on women (if she cleans the bathroom), because it is perceived as violating a principle of gender equality, or because it evokes greater concerns about contamination and impurity among women. The role of disgust may be especially central. Not only does the gender difference in disgust sensitivity account for the greater aversiveness of touching the toilet seat for women, but it may also underlie some of the other theories. Women's fear of falling into the toilet may draw some of its intensity from their greater disgust at the thought of doing so. Their aesthetic preference for a more closed toilet may reflect a desire to reduce its perceived power to contaminate. Their unhappiness about cleaning the bathroom may stem not just from the inequity of a domestic arrangement and from not having caused the mess, but also from the disgustingness of what they are cleaning. Similarly, men's lack of interest in cleaning the bathroom may not only reveal their innate piggishness, but also their failure to see the stray droplets as disgusting to the same degree as women.

Overall, the burden of disgust falls on women more than men. They are held to a higher standard of purity and cleanliness, sanctioned and humiliated more for violating this standard and expected to distance themselves more from the products of their bodies or even to pretend that there are none. In the words of one woman interviewed in a sociological study of 'fecal matters', 'women are supposed to be non-poopers' (Weinberg & Williams, 2005, p. 327). A man in the same study stated that 'women in my mind are beautiful, perfect creatures that are the object of desire... I don't want that image of them tainted in my mind' (p. 327). In a study by Roberts and MacLane described by Goldenberg and Roberts (2004), a female experimenter who excused herself to use the bathroom was evaluated more negatively than one who excused herself to get some paperwork, but no such difference was found for a male experimenter. In addition to being judged more harshly in relation to disgust, women have also often had to do more disgusting work. They have historically borne the brunt of domestic hygiene, including cleaning up the filth of men and children. Sparing women unnecessary disgust should not be too much to ask of men.

So what is to be done? I think it's quite simple: men should put the seat down. Doing so is simple and probably minimizes the overall unpleasantness associated with touching the toilet seat in a mixed-gender household. It eliminates any suspicion of sexism and displays concern for the other person. Men may still enjoy the male prerogative of standing to urinate if they wish, but if they do they should take the lead in cleaning up any resulting splatter. Men may console themselves that in an entirely rational world, in which disgust and contamination concerns were unknown, the self-reliant strategy that many of them prefer would be optimal in terms of efficiency and equity. But they would probably be well advised to console themselves privately or in the exclusive company of men.

References

Abel, E. L., & Buckley, B. E. (1977). *The handwriting on the wall: Toward a sociology and psychology of graffiti*. Westport, CT: Greenwood Press.

Abraham, K. (1917). *Contributions to the theory of the anal character: Selected papers*. London: Hogarth Press.

Abraham, K. (1923). Contributions to the theory of the anal character. *International Journal of Psychoanalysis, 4,* 400–418.

Adorno, T. W., Frenkel-Brunswik, E., Levinson, D. J., & Sanford, R. N. (1950). *The authoritarian personality*. New York: Harper.

Aggarwal, V. R., McBeth, J., Zakrzewska, J. M., Lunt, M., & Macfarlane, G. J. (2006). The epidemiology of chronic syndromes that are frequently unexplained: Do they have common associated factors? *International Journal of Epidemiology, 35,* 468–476.

Ahmed, S. M. (1981). Graffiti of Canadian high-school students. *Psychological Reports, 49,* 559–562.

Alexander, F. (1934). The influence of psychogenic factors upon gastro-intestinal disturbances: a symposium. (1) general principles, objectives, and preliminary results. *Psychoanalytic Quarterly, 3–4,* 501–539.

Alexander, F. (1952). *Psychosomatic medicine: Its principles and applications*. London: George Allen & Unwin.

Alexander, F., & Menninger, W. C. (1936). Relation of persecutory delusions to the functioning of the gastro-intestinal tract. *Journal of Nervous and Mental Disease, 84,* 541.

Alexander, F., & Wilson, G. W. (1936). Quantitative dream studies: A methodological attempt at quantitative evaluation of psychoanalytic material. *Psychoanalytic Quarterly, 4,* 371–407.

Ali, A., Toner, B. B., Stuckless, N., Gallop, R., Diamant, N. E., et al. (2000). Emotional abuse, self-blame, and self-silencing in women with irritable bowel syndrome. *Psychosomatic Medicine, 62,* 76–82.

Allen, V. (2007). *On farting: Language and laughter in the Middle Ages*. New York: Palgrave Macmillan.

American Psychiatric Association (APA) (2000). *Diagnostic and statistical manual of mental disorders* (4th edn, text revision). Washington, DC: APA.

Anderson, S. J., & Verplanck, W. S. (1983). When walls speak, what do they say? *The Psychological Record, 33,* 341–359.

Ansell, E. B., Pinto, A., Crosby, R. D., Becker, D. F., Anez, L. M., Paris, M., & Grilo, C. M. (2010). The prevalence and structure of obsessive-compulsive personality disorder in Hispanic psychiatric outpatients. *Journal of Behavior Therapy and Experimental Psychiatry, 41,* 275–281.

Anthony, K. H., & Dufresne, M. (2007). Potty parity in perspective: Gender and family issues in planning and designing public restrooms. *Journal of Planning Literature, 21*, 267–294.

Appleby, B. S., & Rosenberg, P. B. (2006). Aerophagia as the initial presenting symptom of a depressed patient. *Primacy Care Companion, Journal of Clinical Psychiatry, 8*, 245–246.

Arieti, S. (1944). The 'placing-into-mouth' and coprophagic habits studied from a point of view of comparative developmental psychology. *Journal of Nervous and Mental Disease, 99*, 959–964.

Arluke, A., Kutakoff, L., & Levin, J. (1987). Are the times changing? An analysis of gender differences in sexual graffiti. *Sex Roles, 16*, 1–7.

Arntz, A., Bernstein, D., Gielen, D., van Nieuwenhuijzen, M., Penders, K., Haslam, N., & Ruscio, J. (2009). Taxometric evidence for the dimensional structure of cluster-C, paranoid and borderline personality disorders. *Journal of Personality Disorders, 23*, 606–628.

Ascher, L. M. (1979). Paradoxical intention in the treatment of urinary retention. *Behavior Research and Therapy, 17*, 267–270.

Ashworth, M., Hirdes, J. P., & Martin, L. (2009). The social and recreational characteristics of adults with intellectual disability and pica living in institutions. *Research in Developmental Disabilities, 30*, 512–520.

Baheretibeb, Y., Law, S., & Pain, C. (2008). The girl who ate her house: Pica as an obsessive-compulsive disorder: A case report. *Clinical Case Studies, 7*, 3–11.

Bailey, I. (1961). Pythagoras and the beans. *British Medical Journal, 2 (5253)*, 708–709.

Baker, D. J., Valenzuela, S., & Wieseler, N. A. (2005). Naturalistic inquiry and treatment of coprophagia in one individual. *Journal of Developmental and Physical Disabilities, 17*, 361–367.

Baker, R. (1994). Psychoanalysis as a lifeline: A clinical study of a transference perversion. *The International Journal of Psychoanalysis, 75*, 743–753.

Bansak, C., & Starr, M. (2010). Gender differences in predispositions towards economics. *Eastern Economic Journal, 36*, 33–57.

Bargh, J. A., Chen, M., & Burrows, L. (1996). Automaticity of social behavior: Direct effects of trait construct and stereotype activation on action. *Journal of Personality and Social Psychology, 71*, 230–244.

Barnes, C. (1952). A statistical study of the Freudian theory of levels of psychosexual development. *Genetic Psychology Monographs, 45*, 115–175.

Bartholome, L., & Snyder, P. (2004). Is it philosophy or pornography? Graffiti at the Dinosaur Bar-B-Que. *Journal of American Culture, 27*, 86–98.

Basaran, U. N., Inan, M., Aksu, B., & Ceylan, T. (2007). Colon perforation due to pathologic aerophagia in an intellectually disabled child. *Journal of Paediatrics and Child Health, 43*, 710–712.

Bass, A. (1994). Aspects of urethrality in women. *Psychoanalytic Quarterly, 63*, 491–517.

Bates, J. A., & Martin, M. (1980). The thematic content of graffiti as a non-reactive indicator of male and female attitudes. *Journal of Sex Research, 16*, 300–315.

Beary, M. D., & Cobb, J. P. (1981). Solitary psychosis: Three cases of monosymptomatic delusion of alimentary stench treated with behavioural psychotherapy. *British Journal of Psychiatry, 138*, 64–66.

Beck, D. A., & Frohberg, N. R. (2005). Coprophagia in an elderly man: A case report and review of the literature. *International Journal of Psychiatry in Medicine, 35*, 417–427.

Beckwith, J. B. (1992). Stereotypes and reality in the division of household labor. *Social Behavior and Personality, 20*, 283–288.

Begum, M., & McKenna, P. J. (2011). Olfactory reference syndrome: A systematic review of the world literature. *Psychological Medicine, 41*, 453–461.

Belk, R. W. (1991). The ineluctable mysteries of possessions. *Journal of Social Behavior and Personality, 6*, 17–55.

Beloff, H. (1957). The structure and origin of the anal character. *Genetic Psychology Monographs, 55*, 141–172.

Benarroch, E. (2010). Neural control of the bladder: Recent advances and neurologic implications. *Neurology, 75*, 1839–1846.

Berkeley-Hill, O. (1921). The anal-erotic factor in the religion, philosophy and character of the Hindus. *International Journal of Psychoanalysis, 2*, 306.

Bernstein, A. (1955). Some relations between techniques of feeding and training during infancy and certain behavior in childhood. *Genetic Psychology Monographs, 51*, 3–44.

Bilanakis, N. (2006). Psychogenic urinary retention. *General Hospital Psychiatry, 28*, 259–261.

Bird, J. R. (1980) Psychogenic urinary retention. *Psychotherapy and Psychosomatics, 34*, 45–51.

Birke, L. I., & Sadler, D. (1984). Scent-marking behaviour in response to conspecific odours by the rat, *Rattus norvegicus*. *Animal Behaviour, 32*, 493–500.

Blanchard, E. B., Lackner, J. M., Sanders, K., Krasner, S., Keefer, L., Payne, A., Gudleski, G. D., Katz, L., Rowell, D., Sykes, M., Kuhn, E., Gusmano, R., Carosella, A. M., Firth, R., & Dulgar-Tulloch, L. (2007). A controlled evaluation of group cognitive therapy in the treatment of irritable bowel syndrome. *Behaviour Research and Therapy, 45*, 633–648.

Blankstein, U., Che, J., Diamand, N. E., & Davis, K. D. (2010). Altered brain structure in irritable bowel syndrome: Potential contributions of pre-existing and disease-driven factors. *Gastroenterology, 138*, 1783–1789.

Bogg, T. & Roberts, B. W. (2004). Conscientiousness and health behaviors: A meta-analysis of the leading behavioral contributors to mortality. *Psychological Bulletin, 130*, 887–919.

Boschen, M. J. (2008). Paruresis (psychogenic inhibition of micturition): Cognitive behavioral formulation and treatment. *Depression and Anxiety, 25*, 903–912.

Bowlby, J. (1990). *Charles Darwin: A new biography*. London: Pimlico.

Brill, A. A. (1932). The sense of smell in the neuroses and psychoses. *Psychoanalytic Quarterly, 1*, 7–42.

Brown, N. O. (1968). *Life against death: The psychoanalytical meaning of history*. London: Sphere.

Bruner, E. M., & Kelso, J. P. (1980). Gender differences in graffiti: A semiotic perspective. *Women's Studies International Quarterly, 3*, 239–252.

Burton, R. (1621/1850). *The anatomy of melancholy*. Philadelphia: J. W. Moore.

Buser, M. M., & Ferreira, F. (1980). Models and frequency and content of graffiti. *Perceptual and Motor Skills, 51*, 582.

Bushman, B. J. (2002). Does venting anger feed or extinguish the flame? Catharsis, rumination, distraction, anger, and aggressive responding. *Personality and Social Psychology Bulletin, 28*, 724–731.

Butler, E. (2006). *The anthropology of anonymity: Toilet graffiti and the University of Melbourne*. Research paper 30, School of anthropology, geography and environmental studies, University of Melbourne.

Butler, R. J. (2001). Impact of nocturnal enuresis on children and young people. *Scandinavian Journal of Urology and Nephrology, 35*, 169–176.

Byard, R. W. (2001). Coprophagic café coronary. *American Journal of Forensic Medicine and Pathology, 22*, 96–99.

Cacioppo, J. T., Priester, J. R., & Berntson, G. G. (1993). Rudimentary determination of attitudes: II. Arm flexion and extension have differential effects on attitudes. *Journal of Personality and Social Psychology, 65*, 5–17.

Callaghan, P., Moloney, G., & Blair, D. (2012). Contagion in the representational field of water recycling: Informing new environment practice through social representation theory. *Journal of Community and Applied Social Psychology, 22*, 20–37.

Calloway, S. P., Fonagy, P., & Pounder, R. E., et al. (1983). Behavioral techniques in the management of aerophagia in patients with hiatus hernia. *Journal of Psychosomatic Research, 27*, 499–502.

Case, T. I., Repacholi, B. M., & Stevenson, R. J. (2006). My baby doesn't smell as bad as yours: The plasticity of disgust. *Evolution and Human Behavior, 27*, 357–365.

Chapman, A. H. (1959). Psychogenic urinary retention in women. *Psychosomatic Medicine, 21*, 119–122.

Chapman, L. J., & Chapman, J. P. (1969). Illusory correlation as an obstacle to the use of valid psychodiagnostic signs. *Journal of Abnormal Psychology, 74*, 271–280.

Chaturvedi, S. K. (1988). Coprophagia in a schizophrenic patient: Case report. *Psychopathology, 21*, 31–33.

Cheyne, G. (1733/1976). *The English malady*. Delmar, NY: Scholars' Facsimiles & Reprints.

Chitkara, D. K., Bredenoord, A. J., Rucker, M. J., & Talley, N. J. (2005). Aerophagia in adults: A comparison with functional dyspepsia. *Alimentary Pharmacology & Therapeutics, 22*, 855–858.

Cigrang, J. A., Hunter, C. M., & Peterson, A. L. (2006). Behavioral treatment of chronic belching due to aerophagia in a normal adult. *Behavior Modification, 30*, 341–351.

Cohen, D., Nisbett, R. E., Bowdle, B. F., & Schwartz, N. (1996). Insult, aggression, and the Southern culture of honor: An 'experimental ethnography'. *Journal of Personality and Social Psychology, 70*, 945–960.

Cole, J. A., Rothman, K. J., Cabral, H. J., et al. (2007). Incidence of IBS in a cohort of people with asthma. *Digestive Disease Science, 52*, 329–335.

Coltrane, S. (1989). Household labor and the routine production of gender. *Social Problems, 36*, 473–490.

Coolidge, F. L., Thede, L. L., & Jany, K. J. (2001). Heritability of personality disorders in childhood: A preliminary investigation. *Journal of Personality Disorders, 15*, 33–40.

Costa, P., Samuels, J., Bagby, M., Daffin, L., & Norton, H. (2005). Obsessive-compulsive personality disorder: A review. In M. Maj, H. S. Akiskal, J. E. Mezzich & A. Okasha (eds), *Personality disorders* (pp. 405–439). New York: Norton.

Creed, F., Craig, T., & Farmer, R. (1988). Functional abdominal pain, psychiatric illness, and life events. *Gut, 29*, 235–242.

Cuevas, J. L., Cook, E. W., Richter, J. E., McCutcheon, M., & Taub, E. (1995). Spontaneous swallowing rate and emotional state: Possible mechanism for stress-related gastrointestinal disorders. *Digestive Diseases and Sciences, 40*, 282–286.

Curtis, V., deBarra, M., & Aunger, R. (2011). Disgust as an adaptive system for disease avoidance behaviour. *Philosophical Transactions of the Royal Society B: Biological Sciences, 366*, 389–401.

Davey, G. C. L., Bickerstaffe, S., & MacDonald, B. A. (2006). Experienced disgust causes a negative interpretation bias: A causal role for disgust in anxious psychopathology. *Behaviour Research and Therapy, 44*, 1375–1384.

Davies, G. J., Crowder, M., Reid, B., & Dickerson, J. W. T. (1986). Bowel function measurements of individuals with different eating patterns. *Gut, 27*, 164–169.

Davila, G. W., Bernier, F., Franco, J., & Kopka, S. L. (2003). Bladder dysfunction in sexual abuse survivors. *Journal of Urology, 170*, 476–479.

Denson, R. (1982). Undinism: The fetishization of urine. *Canadian Journal of Psychiatry, 27*, 336–338.

Desmond, A., & Moore, J. (1991). *Darwin: The life of a tormented evolutionist.* New York: Warner Books.

Dewaele, J. (2004). The emotional force of swearwords and taboo words in multilinguals. *Journal of Multilingual & Multicultural Development, 25*, 204–222.

D'Mello, D. (1983). Aerophagia and depression: Case report. *Journal of Clinical Psychiatry, 44*, 387–388.

Dooling, R. (1996). *Blue streak: Swearing, free speech, and sexual harassment.* New York: Random House.

Dorn, S. D., Palsson, O. S., Thiwan, S. I., Kanazawa, M., Clark, W. C., et al. (2007). Increased colonic pain sensitivity in irritable bowel syndrome is the result of an increased tendency to report pain rather than increased neurosensory sensitivity. *Gut, 56*, 1202–1209.

Douglas, M. (1966). *Purity and danger: An analysis of concepts of pollution and taboo*. London: Penguin Books.

Drossman, D. A. (1993). U.S. householder survey of functional gastrointestinal disorders. Prevalence, sociodemography, and health impact. *Digestive Diseases & Sciences, 38*, 1569–1580.

Drossman, D. A., Camilleri, M., Mayer, E. A., et al. (2002). AGA technical review on irritable bowel syndrome. *Gastroenterology, 123*, 2108–2131.

Drossman, D. A., Ringel, Y., Vogt, B. A., Leserman, J., Lin, W., et al. (2003). Alterations of brain activity associated with resolution of emotional distress and pain in a case of severe irritable bowel syndrome. *Gastroenterology, 124*, 754–761.

Druschel, B. A., & Sherman, M. F. (1999). Disgust sensitivity as a function of the Big Five and gender. *Personality and Individual Differences, 26*, 739–748.

Duckitt, J., & Sibley, C. G. (2007). Right wing authoritarianism, social dominance orientation and the dimensions of generalized prejudice. *European Journal of Personality, 21*, 113–130.

Dudley, N. M., Orvis, K. A., Lebiecki, J. E., & Cortina, J. M. (2006). A meta-analytic investigation of Conscientiousness in the prediction of job performance: Examining the intercorrelations and the incremental validity of narrow traits. *Journal of Applied Psychology, 91*, 40–57.

Dunbar, F. (1947). *Mind and body: Psychosomatic medicine*. New York: Random House.

Dundes, A. (1966). Here I sit: A study of American latrinalia. *Kroeber Anthropological Society Papers, 34*, 91–105.

Dundes, A. (1978). Into the endzone for a touchdown: A psychoanalytic consideration of American football. *Western Folklore, 37*, 75–88.

Dundes, A. (1984). *Life is like a chicken coop ladder: A portrait of German culture through folklore*. New York: Columbia University Press.

Durkin, M. S., Khan, N., Davidson, L. L., Zaman, S. S., & Stein, Z. A. (1993). The effects of a natural disaster on child behaviour: Evidence for post-traumatic stress. *American Journal of Public Health, 83*, 1549–1553.

Egan, S. J., Wade, T. D., & Shafran, R. (2011). Perfectionism as a transdiagnostic process: A clinical review. *Clinical Psychology Review, 31*, 203–212.

el-Assra, A. (1987). A case of Gilles de la Tourette's syndrome in Saudi Arabia. *British Journal of Psychiatry, 151*, 397–398.

Elms, A. C. (1977). 'The three bears': Four interpretations. *Journal of American Folklore, 90*, 257–273.

Elsenbruch, S. (2011). Abdominal pain in Irritable Bowel Syndrome: A review of putative psychological, neural and neuro-immune mechanisms. *Brain, Behavior, and Immunity, 25*, 386–394.

Elsenbruch, S., Rosenberger, C., Bingel, U., Forsting, M., Schedlowski, M., & Gizewski, E. R. (2010a). Patients with irritable bowel syndrome have altered modulation of neural responses to visceral stimuli. *Gastroenterology, 139*, 1310–1319.

Elsenbruch, S., Rosenberger, C., Enck, P., Forsting, M., Schedlowski, M., & Gizewski, E. R. (2010b). Affective disturbances modulate the neural processing of visceral pain stimuli in irritable bowel syndrome: An fMRI study. *Gut, 59*, 489–494.

Enck, P., & Klosterhalfen, S. (2005). The placebo response in functional bowel disorders: Perspectives and putative mechanisms. *Neurogastroenterology & Motility, 17*, 325–331.

Enns, M. W., Cox, B. J., & Clara, I. (2002). Adaptive and maladaptive perfectionism: Developmental origins and association with depression proneness. *Personality and Individual Differences, 33*, 921–935.

Erikson, E. H. (1958). *Young man Luther: A study in psychoanalysis and history.* London: Faber.

Erikson, E. H. (1963). *Childhood and society* (2nd edn). New York: Norton.

Etchegoyen, R. H. (2005). *The fundamentals of psychoanalytic technique* (rev. edn). London: Karnac.

Evans, G. W., & Wener, R. E. (2007). Crowding and personal space invasion on the train: Please don't make me sit in the middle. *Journal of Environmental Psychology, 27*, 90–94.

Farr, J. H., & Gordon, C. (1975). A partial replication of Kinsey's graffiti study. *Journal of Sex Research, 11*, 158–162.

Faulkner, J., Schaller, M., Park, J. H., & Duncan, L. A. (2004). Evolved disease-avoidance mechanisms and contemporary xenophobic attitudes. *Group Processes & Intergroup Relations, 7*, 333–353.

Felthous, A. R., & Yudowitz, B. (1977). Approaching a comparative typology of assaultive female offenders. *Psychiatry, 40*, 270–276.

Fenichel, O. (1945). *The psychoanalytic theory of neurosis.* New York: W. W. Norton.

Ferenczi, S. (1950). Flatus as an adult prerogative. In *Further contributions to the theory and teaching of psychoanalysis* (p. 325). London: Hogarth Press.

Fergusson, D. M., Horwood, L. T., & Shannon, F. T. (1990). Secondary enuresis in a birth cohort of New Zealand children. *Paediatrics and Perinatal Epidemiology, 4*, 53–63.

Fishbain, D. A., & Goldberg, M. (1991). Fluoxetine for obsessive fear of loss of control of malodorous flatulence. *Psychosomatics: Journal of Consultation Liaison Psychiatry, 32*, 105–107.

Flaisher, G. F. (1994). The use of suggestion and behavioral methods in the treatment of aerophagia: Two case reports. *Child and Family Behavior Therapy, 16*, 25–32.

Flett, G. L., & Hewitt, P. L. (eds) (2002). *Perfectionism: Theory, research, and treatment.* Washington, DC: American Psychological Association.

Fonagy, P. (1986). The effect of emotional arousal on spontaneous swallowing rates. *Journal of Psychosomatic Research, 30*, 183–188.

Formanek, R. (1991). Why they collect: Collectors reveal their motivations. *Journal of Social Behavior and Personality, 6*, 275–286.

Fowler, C., Griffiths, D., & de Groat, W. C. (2008). The neural control of micturition. *Nature Reviews Neuroscience, 9*, 453–466.

Fraiberg, S. H. (1959). *The magic years: Understanding and handling the problems of early childhood.* New York: Scribner.

Freeman, R. D., Zinner, S. H., Muller-Vahl, K. R., Fast, D. K., Burd, L. J., et al. (2009). Coprophenomena in Tourette syndrome. *Developmental Medicine & Child Neurology, 51*, 218–227.

Freud, S. (1908). Character and anal erotism. In *The Standard Edition of the Complete Psychological Works of Sigmund Freud*, trans. from German under the general editorship of James Strachey, in collaboration with Anna Freud, assisted by Alix Strachey and Alan Tyson, 24 vols (1953–74). London: Hogarth Press and the Institute of Psycho-Analysis, vol. 9. pp. 167–175.

Freud, S. (1930). Civilization and its discontents. In *Standard Edition*, vol. 21, pp. 57–145.

Freud, S. (1932). The acquisition of power over fire. *International Journal of Psychoanalysis, 13*, 405–410.

Freund, K., & Blanchard, R. (1986). The concept of courtship disorder. *Journal of Sex & Marital Therapy, 12*, 79–92.

Frexinos, J., Denis, P., Allemand, H., Allouche, S., Los, F., & Bonnelye, G. (1998). Descriptive study of functional digestive symptoms in the French general population. *Gastroentérologie Clinique et Biologique, 22*, 785–791.

Friedman, M., & Rosenman, R. (1974). *Type A behavior and your heart*. New York: Knopf.

Frink, H. W. (1923). The symbolism of baseball. *International Journal of Psychoanalysis, 4*, 481.

Fromm, E. (1947). *Man for himself*. New York: Rinehart.

Frost, R. O., Heimberg, R. G., Holt, C. S., Mattia, J. I., & Neubauer, A. L. (1993). A comparison of two measures of perfectionism. *Personality and Individual Differences, 14*, 119–126.

Frost, R. O., Steketee, G., & Grisham, J. (2004). Measurement of compulsive hoarding: Saving inventory-revised. *Behaviour Research and Therapy, 42*, 1163–1182.

Frye, R. E., & Hait, E. J. (2006). Air swallowing caused by recurrent ileus in Tourette's syndrome. *Pediatrics, 117*, e1249–e1252.

Furne, J. K., & Levitt, M. D. (1996). Factors influencing frequency of flatus emission by healthy subjects. *Digestive Diseases and Sciences, 41*, 1631–1635.

Gadpaille, W. J. (1974). Graffiti: Psychoanalytic implications. In L. Gross (ed.), *Sexual behavior: Current issues* (pp. 73–83). Flushing, NY: Spectrum.

Galovski, T. E., & Blanchard, E. B. (1998). The treatment of irritable bowel syndrome with hypnotherapy. *Applied Psychophysiology and Biofeedback, 23*, 219–232.

Garamoni, G. L., & Schwartz, R. M. (1986). Type A behavior pattern and compulsive personality: Toward a psychodynamic-behavioral integration. *Clinical Psychology Review, 6*, 311–336.

Garcia, D., Starin, S., & Churchill, R. M. (2001). Treating aerophagia with contingent physical guidance. *Journal of Applied Behavior Analysis, 34*, 89–92.

Ghaziuddin, N., & McDonald, C. (1985). A clinical study of adult coprophagics. *British Journal of Psychiatry, 147*, 312–313.

Giner-Sorolla, R., & Espinosa, P. (2011). Social cuing of guilt by anger and of shame by disgust. *Psychological Science, 22*, 49–53.

Glicklich, L. B. (1951). An historical account of enuresis. *Pediatrics, 8*, 859–876.

Goldenberg, J. L., & Roberts, T. (2004). The beast within the beauty: An existential perspective on the objectification and condemnation of women. In J. Greenberg, S. L. Koole & T. Pyszczynski (eds), *Handbook of experimental existential psychology* (pp. 71–85). New York: Guilford.

Gonos, G. V., Mulkern, V., & Poushinsky, N. (1976). Anonymous expression: A structural view of graffiti. *Journal of American Folklore, 89*, 40–48.

Goodwin, R. D., & Friedman, H. S. (2006). Health status and the five-factor personality traits in a nationally representative sample. *Journal of Health Psychology, 11*, 643–654.

Gorer, G. (1943). Themes in Japanese culture. *Transactions of the New York Academy of Sciences, 2*, 106–124.

Grace, W. J., & Graham, D. T. (1952). Relationship of specific attitudes and emotions to certain bodily diseases. *Psychosomatic Medicine, 14*, 243–251.

Grant, B. F., Hasin, D. S., Stinson, F. S., Dawson, D. A., Chou, S. P., Ruan, W. J., et al. (2004). Prevalence, correlates, and disability of personality disorders in the United States: Results from the national epidemiologic survey on alcohol and related conditions. *Journal of Clinical Psychiatry, 65*, 948–958.

Green, J. A. (2003). The writing on the stall: Gender and graffiti. *Journal of Language and Social Psychology, 22*, 282–296.

Greenstein, F. I. (1965). Personality and political socialization: The theories of authoritarian and democratic character. *Annals of the American Academy of Political and Social Science, 361*, 81–95.

Griffiths, D., Derbyshire, S., Stenger, A., & Resnick, N. (2005). Brain control of normal and overactive bladder. *Journal of Urology, 174*, 1862–1867.

Griffiths, D., & Tadic, S. D. (2008). Bladder control, urgency, and urge incontinence: Evidence from functional brain imaging. *Neurourology and Urodynamics, 27*, 466–474.

Grilo, C. M. (2004). Factor structure of the DSM-IV criteria for obsessive compulsive personality disorder in patients with binge eating disorder. *Acta Psychiatrica Scandinavica, 109*, 64–69.

Grinder, R. E. (1962). Parental childrearing practices, conscience, and resistance to temptation of sixth-grade children. *Child Development, 33*, 803–820.

Groen, J. (1947). Psychogenesis and psychotherapy of ulcerative colitis. *Psychosomatic Medicine, 9*, 151.

Grosser, G. S., & Laczek, W. J. (1963). Prior parochial vs. secular secondary education and utterance latencies to taboo words. *Journal of Psychology, 55*, 263–277.

Gruber, D. L., & Shupe, D. R. (1982). Personality correlates of urinary hesitancy (paruresis) and body shyness in male college students. *Journal of College Student Development, 23*, 308–313.

Grygier, T. G. (1961). *The dynamic personality inventory*. Windsor: NFER.

Gunnarsson, J., & Simrén, M. (2009). Peripheral factors in the pathophysiology of irritable bowel syndrome. *Digestive and Liver Disease, 41*, 788–793.

Gwee, K. A. (2005). Irritable bowel syndrome in developing countries: A disorder of civilization or colonization? *Neurogastroenterology & Motility, 17,* 317–324.

Haidt, J., McCauley, C., & Rozin, P. (1994). Individual differences in sensitivity to disgust: A scale sampling seven domains of disgust elicitors. *Personality and Individual Differences, 16,* 701–713.

Hammelstein, P., Pietrowsky, R., Merbach, M., & Brähler, E. (2005). Psychogenic urinary retention ('paruresis'): Diagnosis and epidemiology in a representative male sample. *Psychotherapy and Psychosomatics, 74,* 308–314.

Hammelstein, P., & Soifer, S. (2006). Is 'shy bladder syndrome' (paruresis) correctly classified as social phobia? *Anxiety Disorders, 20,* 296–311.

Harada, K. I., Yamamoto, K., & Saito, T. (2006). Effective treatment of coprophagia in a patient with schizophrenia with the novel atypical antipsychotic drug perospirone: A case report. *Pharmacopsychiatry, 39,* 113.

Haslam, N., Loughnan, S., & Sun, P. (2011). Beastly: What makes animal metaphors offensive? *Journal of Language and Social Psychology, 30,* 311–325.

Hatterer, J. A., Gorman, J. M., Fyer, A. J., Campeas, R. B., Schneier, F. R., Hollander, E., Papp, L. A., & Liebowitz, M. R. (1990). Pharmacotherapy of four men with paruresis. *American Journal of Psychiatry, 147,* 109–111.

Haug, T. T., Mykletun, A., & Dahl, A. A. (2002). Are anxiety and depression related to gastrointestinal symptoms in the general population? *Scandinavian Journal of Gastroenterology, 37,* 294–298.

Haug, T. T., Mykletun, A., & Dahl, A. A. (2004). The association between anxiety, depression, and somatic symptoms in a large population: The HUNT-II study. *Psychosomatic Medicine, 66,* 845–851.

Hazlett-Stevens, H., Craske, M. G., Mayer, E. A., Chang, L., & Naliboff, B. D. (2003). Prevalence of irritable bowel syndrome among university studies: The roles of worry, neuroticism, anxiety sensitivity and visceral anxiety. *Journal of Psychosomatic Research, 55,* 501–505.

Heath, G. A., Hardesty, V. A., & Goldfine, P. E. (1984). Firesetting, enuresis, and animal cruelty. *Journal of Child and Adolescent Psychotherapy, 1,* 97–100.

Heaton, K. W., Radvan, J., Moutford, R. A., Braddon, F. E. M., & Hughes, A. O. (1992). Defecation frequency and timing, and stool form in the general population. A prospective study. *Gut, 33,* 818–824.

Heim, C., Nater, U. M., Maloney, E., Boneva, R., Jones, J. F., & Reeves, W. C. (2009). Childhood trauma and risk for chronic fatigue syndrome: association with neuroendocrine dysfunction. *Archives of General Psychiatry, 66,* 72–80.

Heimberg, R. G., Holt, C. S., Schneier, F. R., Spitzer, R. L., & Liebowitz, M. R. (1993). The issue of subtypes in the diagnosis of social phobia. *Journal of Anxiety Disorders, 7,* 249–269.

Hellman, D. S., & Blackman, H. (1966). Enuresis, firesetting and cruelty to animals. *American Journal of Psychiatry, 122,* 1431–1435.

Hetherington, E. M., & Brackbill, Y. (1963). Etiology and covariation of obstinacy, orderliness, and parsimony in young children. *Child Development, 34*, 919–943.

Hitschmann, E. (1921). *Freud's theories of the neuroses*. London: Kegan Paul, Trent, Trubner & Co.

Hitschmann, E. (1923). Urethral erotism and obsessional neurosis: Preliminary communication. *International Journal of Psychoanalysis, 4*, 118–119.

Hodson, G., & Costello, K. (2007). Interpersonal disgust, ideological orientations, and dehumanization as predictors of intergroup attitudes. *Psychological Science, 18*, 691–698.

Hoek, H. W. W., & van Hoeken, D. (2003). Review of the prevalence and incidence of eating disorders. *International Journal of Eating Disorders, 34*, 383–396.

Holstege, G. (2005). Micturition and the soul. *Journal of Comparative Neurology, 493*, 15–20.

Houts, A. C. (2000). Fifty years of psychiatric nomenclature: Reflections on the 1943 War Department Technical Bulletin, Medical 203. *Journal of Clinical Psychology, 56*, 935–967.

Howell, S., Poulton, R., Caspi, A., & Talley, N. J. (2003). Relationship between abdominal pain subgroups in the community and psychiatric diagnosis and personality: A birth cohort study. *Journal of Psychosomatic Research, 55*, 179–187.

Hughes, G. (1991). *Swearing: A social history of foul language, oaths and profanity in English*. Oxford: Blackwell.

Hughes, G. (2006). *An encyclopedia of swearing: The social history of oaths, profanity, foul language, and ethnic slurs in the English-speaking world*. Armonk, NY: M. E. Sharpe.

Inbar, Y., Pizarro, D. A., & Bloom, P. (2009a). Conservatives are more easily disgusted than liberals. *Cognition & Emotion, 23*, 714–725.

Inbar, Y., Pizarro, D. A., Knobe, J., & Bloom, P. (2009b). Disgust sensitivity predicts intuitive disapproval of gays. *Emotion, 9*, 435–439.

Innala, S. M., & Ernulf, K. E. (1992). Understanding male homosexual attraction: An analysis of restroom graffiti. *Journal of Social Behavior and Personality, 7*, 503–510.

Jackson, J. A., & Salisbury, H. M. (1922). *Outwitting our nerves: A primer of psychotherapy*. New York: The Century Co.

Jaffe, M. E., & Sharma, K. K. (1998). Malingering uncommon psychiatric symptoms among defendants charged under California's 'Three Strikes and You're Out' law. *Journal of Forensic Sciences, 43*, 549–555.

Jankovic, J. (2007). Tics and Tourette's syndrome. In J. Jankovic & E. Tolosa (eds), *Parkinson's disease and movement disorders* (5th edn), (pp. 356–375). Philadelphia: Lippincott Williams & Wilkins.

Jay, T. (1992). *Cursing in America: A psycholinguistic study of dirty language in the courts, in the movies, in the schoolyards and on the streets*. Philadelphia and Amsterdam: John Benjamins.

Jay, T. (2000). *Why we curse*. Philadelphia: John Benjamins.

Jay, T., & Janschewitz, K. (2008). The pragmatics of swearing. *Journal of Politeness Research, 4*, 267–288.

Jay, T., King, K., & Duncan, T. (2006). College students' memories of punishment for cursing. *Sex Roles, 55*, 123–133.

Jones, E. (1918). Analytic study of a case of obsessional neurosis. In *Papers on psychoanalysis* (pp. 515–539). Baltimore: William Wood & Company.

Jones, E. (1918/1950). Anal-erotic character traits. In *Papers on psychoanalysis* (5th edn), (pp. 413–437). London: Baillière, Tindall & Cox.

Jones, E. (1964). *The life and work of Sigmund Freud* (abridged edn). London: Pelican.

Jones, J. H. (1997). *Alfred C. Kinsey: A public/private life*. New York: W. W. Norton.

Judge, T. A., Higgins, C. A., Thoresen, C. J., & Barrick, M. R. (1999). The big five personality traits, general mental ability, and career success across the life span. *Personnel Psychology, 52*, 621–652.

Jung, C. G. (1963). *Memories, dreams, reflections* (rev. edn). New York: Pantheon.

Juni, S. (1984). The psychodynamics of disgust. *Journal of Genetic Psychology, 144*, 203–208.

Kanaan, R. A. A., Lepine, J. P., & Wessely, S. C. (2007). The association or otherwise of the functional somatic syndromes. *Psychosomatic Medicine, 69*, 855–859.

Kaplan, R. M. (2010). Freud's excellent adventure Down Under: The only publication in Australia by the founder of psychoanalysis. *Australasian Psychiatry, 18*, 205–209.

Keefer, L., & Blanchard, E. B. (2001). The effects of relaxation response meditation on the symptoms of irritable bowel syndrome: Results of a controlled treatment study. *Behaviour Research and Therapy, 39*, 801–811.

Kern, M. L., & Friedman, H. S. (2008). Do conscientious people live longer? A quantitative review. *Health Psychology, 27*, 505–512.

Kessler, M. M., & Poucher, G. E. (1945). Coprophagy in the absence of insanity: A case report. *Journal of Nervous and Mental Disease, 102*, 290–293.

Kiesling, S. F. (1998). Men's identities and sociolinguistic variation: The case of fraternity men. *Journal of Sociolinguistics, 2*, 69–99.

Kinsey, A. C., Pomeroy, W. B., Martin, C. E., & Gebhard, P. H. (1953). *Sexual behavior in the human female*. Philadelphia: W. B. Saunders.

Kipfer, B. A., & Chapman, R. L. (2007). *Dictionary of American slang* (4th edn). New York: Collins.

Kline, P. (1968). The validity of the Dynamic Personality Inventory. *British Journal of Medical Psychology, 41*, 307–311.

Kline, P. (1969). The anal character: A cross-cultural study in Ghana. *British Journal of Social and Clinical Psychology, 8*, 201–210.

Kline, P., & Cooper, C. (1984). Factorial analysis of the authoritarian character. *British Journal of Psychology, 75*, 171–176.

Koocher, G. P. (1977). Bathroom behavior and human dignity. *Journal of Personality and Social Psychology, 35*, 120–121.

Kotthoff, H. (2006). Gender and humor: The state of the art. *Journal of Pragmatics, 38*, 4–25.

Krugman, R. D. (1984). Fatal child abuse: Analysis of 24 cases. *Pediatrician, 12*, 68–72.

Kubie, L. S. (1937). The fantasy of dirt. *Psychoanalytic Quarterly, 6*, 388–425.

Kubota, F. (1987). A case of automysophobia treated by JIKO-control method. *Japanese Journal of Hypnosis, 32*, 27–33.

Kurlan, R., Daragjati, C., Como, P. G., McDermott, M. P., Trinidad, K. S., Roddy, S., Brower, C. A., & Robertson, M. M. (1996). Non-obscene complex socially inappropriate behavior in Tourette's syndrome. *Journal of Neuropsychiatry and Clinical Neurosciences, 8*, 311–317.

Kushner, H. I. (1999). *A cursing brain? The histories of Tourette syndrome*. Cambridge, MA: Harvard University Press.

Lackner, J. M., Brasel, A. M., Quigley, B. M., Keefer, L., Krasner, S. S., Powell, C., Katz, L. A., & Sitrin, M. D. (2010). The ties that bind: Perceived social support, stress, and IBS in severely affected patients. *Neurogastroenterology & Motility, 22*, 893–900.

Lackner, J. M., & Gurtman, M. B. (2000). Patterns of interpersonal problems in irritable bowel syndrome: A circumplex analysis. *Journal of Psychosomatic Research, 58*, 523–532.

Ladas, S. D., Karamanolis, G., & Ben-Soussan, E. (2007). Colonic gas explosion during therapeutic colonoscopy with electrocautery. *World Journal of Gastroenterology, 13(40)*, 5295–5298.

Ladouceur, R., Freeston, M. H., Gagnon, F., Thibodeau, N., & Dumont, J. (1993). Idiographic considerations in the behavioral treatment of obsessional thoughts. *Journal of Behavior Therapy and Experimental Psychiatry, 24*, 301–310.

Lakoff, R. (1975). *Language and women's place*. New York: Harper & Row.

Landy, E. E., & Steele, J. M. (1967). Graffiti as a function of building utilization. *Perceptual and Motor Skills, 25*, 711–712.

Lang, A., Consky, E., & Sandor, P. (1993). 'Signing tics': Insights into the pathophysiology of symptoms in Tourette's syndrome. *Annals of Neurology, 33*, 212–215.

Lang, M. L. (1988). *Graffiti in the Athenian agora*. Meriden, CT: Meriden-Stinehour Press.

Langendorfer, F. (2008). Personality differences among orchestra instruments: Just a stereotype? *Personality and Individual Differences, 44*, 610–620.

Lazare, A., Klerman, G. L., & Armor, D. J. (1966). Oral, obsessive, and hysterical personality patterns. *Archives of General Psychiatry, 14*, 624–630.

Lerner, B. (1961). Auditory and visual thresholds for the perception of words of anal connotation: An evaluation of the 'sublimation hypothesis' on philatelists. Unpublished doctoral dissertation, Ferkauf Graduate School of Education, Yeshiva University, New York.

Leroy, A. (1929). Coprophagie de nature anxieuse. *Journal de Neurologie et de Psychiatrie, 6*, 339–342.

Levine, J. M., & McBurney, D. H. (1986). The role of olfaction in social perception and behavior. In P. Herman, M. P. Zanna & E. T. Higgins (eds), *Physical appearance, stigma, and social behavior: The Ontario symposium*, vol. 3 (pp. 179–217). Mahwah, NJ: Lawrence Erlbaum.

Levitt, M. D. (1980). Intestinal gas production: Recent advances in flatology. *New England Journal of Medicine, 302*, 1474–1475.

Levitt, M. D., Furne, J., Aeolus, M. R., & Suarez, F. L. (1998). Evaluation of an extremely flatulent patient: Case report and proposed diagnostic and therapeutic approach. *American Journal of Gastroenterology, 93*, 2276–2281.

Levy, R. L., Cain, K. C., Jarrett, M., et al. (1997). The relationship between daily life stress and gastrointestinal symptoms in women with irritable bowel syndrome. *Journal of Behavioral Medicine, 20*, 177–193.

Levy, R. L., Jones, K. R., Whitehead, E. E., et al. (2001). Irritable bowel syndrome in twins: Heredity and social learning both contribute to etiology. *Gastroenterology, 121*, 799–804.

Levy, R. L., Olden, K. W., Naliboff, B., et al. (2006). Psychosocial aspects of the functional gastrointestinal disorders. *Gastroenterology, 130*, 1447–1458.

Link, C. L., Lutfey, K. E., Steers, W. D., & McKinlay, J. B. (2007). Is abuse causally related to urologic symptoms? Results from the Boston Area Community Health (BACH) survey. *European Urology, 52*, 397–406.

Lippman, L. G. (1980). Toward a social psychology of flatulence: The interpersonal regulation of natural gas. *Psychology: A Journal of Human Behavior, 17*, 41–50.

Ljung, M. (2011). *Swearing: A cross-cultural linguistic study*. London: Palgrave Macmillan.

Loewenstine, H. V., Ponticos, G. D., & Paludi, M. A. (1982). Sex differences in graffiti as a communication style. *Journal of Social Psychology, 117*, 307–308.

Lomas, H. D. (1973). Graffiti: Some observations and speculations. *The Psychoanalytic Review, 60*, 71–89.

Lomas, H. D. (1976). Graffiti: Some clinical observations. *The Psychoanalytic Review, 63*, 451–457.

Lomas, H. D. (1980). Graffiti: Additional clinical observations. *The Psychoanalytic Review, 67*, 139–142.

London, L. S. (1950). The psychogenesis of urolagnia in a case of multiple paraphilias. In L. S. London & F. Caprio, *Sexual deviations* (pp. 576–587). Washington, DC: Linacre Press.

Longenecker, G. J. (1977). Sequential parody graffiti. *Western Folklore, 36*, 354–364.

Longstreth, G. F., & Yao, J. F. (2004). Irritable bowel syndrome and surgery: A multivariable analysis. *Gastroenterology, 126*, 1665–1673.

Lorand, S. (1931). Aggression and flatus. *International Journal of Psychoanalysis, 12*, 368.

Lown, E. A., & Vega, W. A. (2001). Intimate partner violence and health: Self-assessed health, chronic health, and somatic symptoms among Mexican American women. *Psychosomatic Medicine, 63*, 352–360.

Lucca, N., & Pacheco, A. M. (1986). Children's graffiti: Visual communication from a developmental perspective. *Journal of Genetic Psychology, 147,* 465–479.

Luciano, M., Wainwright, M. A., & Martin, N. G. (2006). The heritability of conscientiousness facets and their relationship to IQ and academic achievement. *Personality and Individual Differences, 40,* 1189–1199.

Luxem, M., & Christophersen, E. (1994). Behavioral toilet training in early childhood: Research, practice, and implications. *Developmental and Behavioral Pediatrics, 15,* 370–378.

Lyketsos, C. G. (1992). Successful treatment of bowel obsessions with nortriptyline. *The American Journal of Psychiatry, 149,* 573.

Lynam, D., & Widiger, T. (2001). Using the five-factor model to represent the DSM-IV personality disorders: An expert consensus approach. *Journal of Abnormal Psychology, 110,* 401–412.

Malouff, J. M., & Lanyon, R. I. (1985). Avoidant paruresis: An exploratory study. *Behavior Modification, 9,* 225–234.

Mariwah, S., & Drangert, J-O. (2011). Community perceptions of human excreta as fertilizer in peri-urban agriculture in Ghana. *Waste Management & Research, 29,* 815–822.

Marks, I. M. (1987). *Fears, phobias, and rituals: Panic, anxiety, and their disorders.* Oxford University Press.

Martens, U., et al. (2010). Motivation for psychotherapy in patients with functional gastrointestinal disorders. *Psychosomatics, 51,* 225–229.

Martin, J. A., King, D. R., Maccoby, E. E., & Jacklin, C. N. (1984). Secular trends and individual differences in toilet-training progress. *Journal of Pediatric Psychology, 9,* 457–467.

Martin, R. A., Puhlik-Doris, P., Larsen, G., Gray, J., & Weir, K. (2003). Individual differences in the uses of humor and their relation to psychological well-being: Development of the Humor Styles Questionnaire. *Journal of Research in Personality, 37,* 48–75.

Mayer, B., Muris, P., Busser, K., & Bergamin, J. (2009). A disgust mood state causes negative interpretation bias, but not in the specific domain of body-related concerns. *Behaviour Research and Therapy, 47,* 876–881.

McCann, C., Duckworth, A. L., & Roberts, R. D. (2009). Empirical identification of the major facets of Conscientiousness. *Learning and Individual Differences, 19,* 451–458.

McClelland, D. C., & Pilon, D. A. (1983). Sources of adult motives in patterns of parent behavior in early childhood. *Journal of Personality and Social Psychology, 44,* 564–574.

McCracken, L. M., & Larkin, K. T. (1991). Treatment of paruresis with *in vivo* desensitization: A case report. *Journal of Behavior Therapy and Experimental Psychiatry, 22,* 57–63.

McCrae, R. R., & Costa, P. T. (1987). Validation of the five-factor model of personality across instruments and observers. *Journal of Personality and Social Psychology, 52,* 81–90.

McEnery, T. (2005). *Swearing in English: Bad language, purity and power from 1586 to the present*. Abingdon: Routledge.

McGee, M. D., & Gutheil, T. G. (1989). Coprophagia and urodipsia in a chronic mentally ill woman. *Hospital & Community Psychiatry, 40*, 302–303.

McIntosh, W. D., & Schmeichel, B. (2004). Collectors and collecting: A social psychological perspective. *Leisure Sciences, 26*, 85–97.

McMenemy, P., & Cornish, I. M. (1993). Gender differences in the judged acceptability of graffiti. *Perceptual and Motor Skills, 77*, 622.

Merrill, B. R. (1951). Childhood attitudes toward flatulence and their possible relation to adult character. *The Psychoanalytic Quarterly, 20*, 550–564.

Mertz, H., Naliboff, B., Munakata, J., Niazi, N., & Mayer, E. A. (1995). Altered rectal perception is a biological marker of patients with irritable bowel syndrome. *Gastroenterology, 109*, 40–52.

Middlemist, R. D., Knowles, E. S., & Matter, C. F. (1976). Personal space invasions in the lavatory: Suggestive evidence for arousal. *Journal of Personality and Social Psychology, 33*, 541–546.

Milan, M. A., & Kolko, D. J. (1982). Paradoxical intention in the treatment of obsessional flatulence ruminations. *Journal of Behavior Therapy and Experimental Psychiatry, 13*, 167–172.

Montagu, A. (1967). *The anatomy of swearing*. London and New York: Macmillan & Collier.

Motley, M. T., & Camden, C. T. (1985). Nonlinguistic influences on lexical selection: Evidence from double entendres. *Communication Monographs, 52*, 124–135.

Nataskin, I., Mehdikhani, E., Conklin, J. et al. (2006). Studying the overlap between IBS and GERD: A systematic review of the literature. *Digestive Disease Science, 51*, 2113–2120.

Nicholl, B. I., Halder, S. L., Macfarlane, G. J., et al. (2008). Psychosocial risk markers for new onset irritable bowel syndrome: Results of a large prospective population-based study. *Pain, 137*, 147–155.

Niedenthal, P., Barsalou, L. W., Winkielman, P., Krauth-Gruber, S., & Ric, F. (2005). Embodiment in attitudes, social perception, and emotion. *Personality and Social Psychology Review, 9*, 184–211.

Nierenberg, J. (1994). Proverbs in graffiti: Taunting traditional wisdom. In W. Mieder (ed.), *Wise words: Essays on the proverb* (pp. 543–562). New York: Garland.

Nisbett, R. E., & Masuda, T. (2003). Culture and point of view. *Proceedings of the National Academy of Sciences, 100*, 11163–11170.

Nour, S., Svarer, C., Kristensen, J. K., Paulson, O. B., & Law, I. (2000). Cerebral activation during micturition in normal men. *Brain, 123*, 781–789.

Nozu, T., Kudaira, M., Kitamori, S., & Uehara, A. (2006). Repetitive rectal painful distension induces rectal hypersensitivity in patients with irritable bowel syndrome. *Journal of Gastroenterology, 41*, 217–222.

Nussbaum, M. C. (2004). *Hiding from humanity: Disgust, shame, and the law*. Princeton University Press.

Nwoye, O. G. (1993). Social issues of walls: Graffiti in university lavatories. *Discourse & Society, 4*, 419–442.

Oaten, M., Stevenson, R. J., & Case, T. I. (2009). Disgust as a disease avoidance mechanism. *Psychological Bulletin, 135*, 303–321.

O'Donnell, L. J. D., Virjee, J., & Heaton, K. W. (1990). Detection of pseudodiarrhoea by simple clinical assessment of intestinal transit rate. *British Medical Journal, 300*, 439–440.

Olatunji, B. O., Moretz, M. W., McKay, D., Bjorklund, F., de Jong, P. J., Haidt, J., et al. (2009). Conforming the three-factor structure of the Disgust Scale-Revised in eight countries. *Journal of Cross-Cultural Psychology, 40*, 234–255.

Olatunji, B. O., Williams, N. L., Tolin, D. F., Sawchuk, C. N., Abramowitz, J. S., Lohr, J. M., et al. (2007). The Disgust Scale: Item analysis, factor structure, and suggestions for refinement. *Psychological Assessment, 19*, 281–297.

Olowu, A. A. (1983). Graffiti here and there. *Psychological Reports, 52*, 986.

Orlansky, H. (1949). Infant care and personality. *Psychological Bulletin, 46*, 1–48.

Ortner, S. (1972). Is female to male and nature is to culture? *Feminist Studies, 1*, 5–31.

Otta, E., Santana, P. R., Lafraia, L. M., Hoshino, R. L., Teixeira, R. P., & Vallochi, S. L. (1996). Musa latrinalis: Gender differences in restroom graffiti. *Psychological Reports, 78*, 871–880.

Pakhomou, S. M. (2006). Methodological aspects of telephone scatologia: A case study. *International Journal of Law and Psychiatry, 29*, 178–185.

Papolos, D., Hennen, J., & Cockerham, M. S. (2005). Factors associated with parent-reported suicide threats by children and adolescents with community-diagnosed bipolar disorder. *Journal of Affective Disorders, 86*, 267–275.

Peretti, P. O., Carter, R., & McClinton, B. (1977). Graffiti and adolescent personality. *Adolescence, 12*, 31–42.

Perona, M., Benasayag, R., Perello, A., et al. (2005). Prevalence of functional gastrointestinal disorders in women who report domestic violence to the police. *Clinical Gastroenterology and Hepatology, 3*, 436–441.

Persons, J. B., & Foa, E. (1984). Processing of fearful and neutral information for obsessive-compulsives. *Behaviour Research and Therapy, 22*, 259–265.

Pettit, T. (1969). Anality and time. *Journal of Consulting and Clinical Psychology, 33*, 170–174.

Pierce, J. L., Kostova, T., & Dirks, K. T. (2003). The state of psychological ownership: Integrating and extending a century of research. *Review of General Psychology, 7*, 84–107.

Poirel, N., Pineau, A., Jobard, G., & Mellet, E. (2008). Seeing the forest before the trees depends on individual field-dependence characteristics. *Experimental Psychology, 55*, 328–333.

Prüss-Üstün, A., Bos, R., Gore, F., & Bartram, J. (2008). *Safer water, better health: Costs, benefits and sustainability of interventions to protect and promote health.* Geneva: World Health Organization.

Rabelais, F. (1564/1965). *The histories of Gargantua and Pantagruel*. London: Penguin.

Razali, S. M. (1998). Schizophrenia and consuming body waste. *Australian and New Zealand Journal of Psychiatry, 32*, 888–890.

Read, A. W. (1935). *Lexical evidence from folk epigraphy in western North American, a glossarial study of the low elements in the English language*. Paris: Olympic Press.

Reed, G. F. (1985). *Obsessional experience and compulsive behavior: A cognitive-structural approach*. Orlando, FL: Academic Press.

Rees, B., & Leach, D. (1975). The social inhibition of micturition (paruresis): Sex similarities and differences. *Journal of the American College Health Association, 23*, 203–205.

Reich, W. (1933/1949). *Character analysis*. New York: Orgone Institute Press.

Reichborn-Kjennerud, T., Czajkowski, N., Neale, M. C., et al. (2007). Genetic and environmental influences on dimensional representations of DSM-IV cluster C personality disorders: A population-based multivariate twin study. *Psychological Medicine, 37*, 645–653.

Reiskel, K. (1906). Skatologische inschriften. *Anthropophyteia, 3*, 244–246.

Rey, E., & Talley, N. J. (2009). Irritable bowel syndrome: Novel views on the epidemiology and potential risk factors. *Digestive and Liver Disease, 41*, 772–780.

Reynolds, C., & Haslam, N. (2011). Evidence for an association between women and nature: An analysis of media images and mental representations. *Ecopsychology, 3*, 59–64.

Riedl, A., et al. (2008). Somatic comorbidities of irritable bowel syndrome: A systematic analysis. *Journal of Psychosomatic Research, 64*, 573–582.

Ringel, Y., Drossman, D. A., Leserman, J. L., Suyenobu, B. Y., Wilber, K., et al. (2008). Effect of abuse history on pain reports and brain responses to aversive visceral stimulation: An fMRI study. *Gastroenterology, 134*, 396–404.

Robbins, J. M., Kirmayer, L. J., & Hemami, S. (1997). Latent variable models of functional somatic distress. *Journal of Nervous and Mental Disease, 185*, 606–615.

Roberts, B. W., & Bogg, T. (2004). A 30-year longitudinal study of the relationships between conscientiousness-related traits, and the family structure and health-behavior factors that affect health. *Journal of Personality, 72*, 325–354.

Roberts, B. W., Kuncel, N. R., Shiner, R., Caspi, A., & Goldberg, L. R. (2007). The power of personality: The comparative validity of personality traits, socioeconomic status, and cognitive ability for predicting important life outcomes. *Perspectives on Psychological Science, 2*, 313–345.

Rodriguez, A. J., Holleran, S. E., & Mehl, M. R. (2010). Reading between the lines: The lay assessment of subclinical depression from written self-descriptions. *Journal of Personality, 78*, 575–597.

Roheim, G. (1934). The study of character development and the ontogenetic theory of culture. In E. E. Evans-Pritchard, R. Firth, B. Malinowski & I. Schapera (eds), *Essays presented to C. G. Seligman* (pp. 281–291). London: Kegan Paul, Trench, Hubner & Co.

Rosenbaum, R. (1998). *Explaining Hitler: The search for the origin of his evil.* New York: Random House.
Rosenberger, C., Elsenbruch, S., Scholle, A., De Greiff, A., Schedlowski, M., Forsting, M., & Gizewski, E. R. (2009). Effects of psychological stress on the cerebral processing of visceral stimuli in healthy women. *Neurogastroenterology & Motility, 21,* 740–e45.
Rosenquist, L. E. D. (2005). A psychosocial analysis of the human-sanitation nexus. *Journal of Environmental Psychology, 25,* 335–346.
Rosenwald, G. C., Mendelson, G. A., Fontana, A., & Portz, A. T. (1966). An action test of hypotheses concerning the anal personality. *Journal of Abnormal Psychology, 71,* 304–309.
Rozin, P. (2006). Domain denigration and process preference in academic psychology. *Perspectives in Psychological Science, 1,* 365–376.
Rozin, P. (2007). Exploring the landscape of modern academic psychology: Finding and filling the holes. *American Psychologist, 62,* 754–766.
Rozin, P., & Fallon, A. E. (1987). A perspective on disgust. *Psychological Review, 94,* 23–41.
Rozin, P., Haidt, J., & Fincher, K. (2009). From oral to moral. *Science, 323,* 1179–1180.
Rozin, P., Hammer, L., Oster, H., Horowitz, T., & Marmora, V. (1986). The child's conception of food: Differentiation of categories of rejected food in the 1.4 to 5 year range. *Appetite, 7,* 141–151.
Saito, Y. A., Schoenfeld, P., & Locke, G. R., III (2002). The epidemiology of irritable bowel syndrome in North America: A systematic review. *American Journal of Gastroenterology, 97,* 1910–1915.
Sakamaki, T. (2010). Coprophagy in wild bonobos (*Pan paniscus*) at Wamba in the Democratic Republic of Congo: A possible adaptive strategy? *Primates, 51,* 87–90.
Samuel, D. B., & Widiger, T. A. (2011). Conscientiousness and obsessive-compulsive personality disorder. *Personality Disorders: Theory, Research, and Treatment, 2,* 161–174.
Schaller, M., & Murray, D. R. (2008). Pathogens, personality, and culture: Disease prevalence predicts worldwide variability in sociosexuality, extraversion, and openness to experience. *Journal of Personality and Social Psychology, 95,* 212–221.
Schlachter, A., & Duckitt, J. (2002). Psychopathology, authoritarian attitudes, and prejudice. *South African Journal of Psychology, 32,* 1–8.
Schnall, S., Haidt, J., Clore, G. L., & Jordan, A. H. (2008). Disgust as embodied moral judgment. *Personality and Social Psychology Bulletin, 34,* 1096–1109.
Schreer, G. E., & Strichartz, J. M. (1997). Private restroom graffiti: An analysis of controversial social issues on two college campuses. *Psychological Reports, 81,* 1067–1074.
Schroeder, S. R. (1989). Rectal digging, feces smearing, and coprophagy. In T. B. Karasu (ed.), *Treatment of psychiatric disorders,* vol. 1 (pp. 43–44). Washington, DC: American Psychiatric Association.

Schwartz, M. J., & Dovidio, J. F. (1984). Reading between the lines: Personality correlates of graffiti writing. *Perceptual and Motor Skills, 59*, 395–398.

Schwarz, S. P., Taylor, A. E., Scharff, L., & Blanchard, E. B. (1990). Behaviorally treated Irritable Bowel Syndrome patients: A four-year follow-up. *Behaviour Research and Therapy, 28*, 331–335.

Sears, R. R. (1936). Studies of projection: I. Attribution of traits. *Journal of Social Psychology, 7*, 151–163.

Sechrest, L., & Flores, L. (1969). Homosexuality in Philippines and United States: Handwriting on wall. *Journal of Social Psychology, 79*, 3–12.

Sechrest, L., & Olson, A. K. (1971). Graffiti in four types of institutions of higher education. *Journal of Sex Research, 7*, 62–71.

Semin, G. R., & Rubini, M. (1990). Unfolding the concept of person through verbal abuse. *European Journal of Social Psychology, 20*, 463–474.

Sewell, W. H., Mussen, P. H., & Harris, C. W. (1955). Relationships among child training practices. *American Sociological Review, 20*, 137–148.

Shapiro, D. (1965). *Neurotic styles*. New York: Basic Books.

Sibley, C. G., & Duckitt, J. (2008). Personality and prejudice: A meta-analysis and theoretical review. *Personality and Social Psychology Review, 12*, 248–279.

Sidoli, M. (1996). Farting as a defence against unspeakable dread. *Journal of Analytical Psychology, 41*, 165–178.

Simkin, B. (1992). Mozart's scatological disorder. *British Medical Journal, 305*, 1563–1567.

Singer, C. (1997). Tourette syndrome: Coprolalia and other coprophenomena. *Neurological Clinics, 15*, 299–308.

Singer, H. S. (2000). Current issues in Tourette syndrome. *Movement Disorders, 15*, 1051–1063.

Smith, R. A., Farnworth, H., Wright, B., & Allgar, V. (2009). Are there more bowel symptoms in children with autism compared to normal children and children with other developmental and neurological disorders? A case control study. *Autism, 13*, 343–355.

Snel, J., Burgering, M., Smit, B., Noordman, W., Tangerman, A., Winkel, E. G., & Kleerebezem, M. (2011). Volatile sulphur compounds in morning breath of human volunteers. *Archives of Oral Biology, 56*, 29–34.

Solomon, H., & Yager, H. (1975). Authoritarianism and graffiti. *Journal of Social Psychology, 97*, 149–150.

Sperling, M. (1948). Diarrhea: A specific somatic equivalent of an unconscious emotional conflict. *Psychosomatic Medicine, 10*, 331–334.

Stenner, P. H. D., Dancey, C. P., & Watts, S. (2000). The understanding of their illness amongst people with irritable bowel syndrome: A Q methodological study. *Social Science & Medicine, 51*, 439–452.

Stephens, R., Atkins, J., & Kingston, A. (2009). Swearing as a response to pain. *NeuroReport, 20*, 1056–1060.

Stocker, T. L., Dutcher, L. W., Hargrove, S. M., & Cook, E. (1972). Social analysis of graffiti. *Journal of American Folklore, 85*, 356–366.

Stoeber, J., & Otto, K. (2006). Positive conceptions of perfectionism: Approaches, evidence, challenges. *Personality and Social Psychology Review, 10*, 295–319.

Strachey, J. (1930). Some unconscious factors in reading. *The International Journal of Psychoanalysis, 11*, 322–331.

Strack, F., Martin, L. L., & Steper, S. (1988). Inhibiting and facilitating conditions of the human smile: A nonobtrusive test of the facial feedback hypothesis. *Journal of Personality and Social Psychology, 54*, 768–777.

Strömgren, A., & Thomsen, P. H. (1990). Personality traits in young adults with a history of conditioning-treated childhood enuresis. *Acta Psychiatrica Scandinavica, 81*, 538–541.

Suarez, F. L., Furne, J. K., Springfield, J., & Levitt, M. D. (2000). Morning breath odor: Influence of treatments on sulfur gases. *Journal of Dental Research, 79*, 1773–1777.

Suarez, F. L., Springfield, J., & Levitt, M. D. (1998). Identification of gases responsible for the odour of human flatus and evaluation of a device purported to reduce this odour. *Gut, 43*, 100–104.

Szasz, T. S. (1951). Physiologic and psychodynamic mechanisms in constipation and diarrhea. *Psychosomatic Medicine, 13*, 112–116.

Talley, N. J., Boyce, P. M., & Jones, M. (1998). Is the association between irritable bowel syndrome and abuse explained by neuroticism? A population based study. *Gut*, 42, 47–53.

Talley, N. J., Dennis, E. H., Schettler-Duncan, V. A. et al. (2003). Overlapping upper and lower gastrointestinal symptoms in irritable bowel syndrome patients with constipation or diarrhea. *American Journal of Gastroenterology, 98*, 2454–2459.

Talley, N. J., Fett, S. L., Zinsmeister, A. R., et al. (1994). Gastrointestinal tract symptoms and self-reported abuse: A population-based study. *Gastroenterology, 107*, 1040–1049.

Talley, N. J., Fett, S. L., & Zinsmeister, A. R. (1995). Self-reported abuse and gastrointestinal disease in outpatients: Association with irritable bowel-type symptoms. *American Journal of Gastroenterology, 90*, 366–371.

Tangney, J. P., & Dearing, R. L. (2002). *Shame and guilt*. New York: Guilford.

Tangney, J. P., Miller, R. S., Flicker, L., & Barlow, D. H. (1996). Are shame, guilt, and embarrassment distinct emotions? *Journal of Personality and Social Psychology, 70*, 1256–1269.

Templer, D. I., King, F. L., Brooner, R. K., & Corgiat, M. (1984). Assessment of body elimination attitude. *Journal of Clinical Psychology, 40*, 754–759.

Thornhill, R., Fincher, C. L., & Aran, D. (2009). Parasites, democratization, and the liberalization of values across contemporary countries. *Biological Reviews, 84*, 113–131.

Thrumbo, H. (1731). *The merry-thought: or, the glass-window and bog-house miscellany*. London.

Tolin, D. F., Woods, C. M., & Abramowitz, J. S. (2006). Disgust sensitivity and obsessive-compulsive symptoms in a nonclinical sample. *Journal of Behavior Therapy and Experimental Psychiatry, 37*, 30–40.

Tuk, M. A., Trampe, D., & Warlop, L. (2011). Inhibitory spillover: Increased urination urgency facilitates impulse control in unrelated domains. *Psychological Science, 22,* 627–633.

Turk, C. L., Heimberg, R. G., Orsillo, S. M., Holt, C. S., Gitow, A., Street, L. L., Schneier, E. R., & Liebowitz, M. R. (1998). An investigation of gender differences in social phobia. *Journal of Anxiety Disorders, 12,* 209–223.

Vaes, J., Paladino, M., & Puvia, E. (2011). Are sexualized women complete human beings? Why men and women dehumanize sexually objectified women. *European Journal of Social Psychology, 41,* 774–785.

Van der Kolk, M. B. (1999). Acute abdomen in mentally retarded patients: Role of aerophagia. Report on nine cases. *European Journal of Surgery, 165,* 507–511.

Van Haarst, E. P., Heldeweg, E. A., Newling, D. W., & Schlatmann, T. J. (2004). The 24-h frequency-volume chart in adults reporting no voiding complaints: Defining reference values and analysing variables. *BJU International, 93,* 1257–1261.

Van Hiel, A., Mervielde, I., & De Fruyt, F. (2004a). The relationship between maladaptive personality and right wing ideology. *Personality and Individual Differences, 36,* 405–417.

Van Hiel, A., Pandelaere, M., & Duriez, B. (2004b). The impact of need for closure on conservative beliefs and racism: Differential mediation by authoritarian submission and authoritarian dominance. *Personality and Social Psychology Bulletin, 30,* 824–837.

Van Hoecke, E., De Fruyt, F., De Clerq, B., Hoebeke, P., & Vander Walle, J. (2006). Internalizing and externalizing problem behavior in children with nocturnal and diurnal enuresis: A five-factor model perspective. *Journal of Pediatric Psychology, 31,* 460–468.

Van Lancker, D., & Cummings, J. L. (1999). Expletives: Neurolinguistics and neurobehavioral perspectives on swearing. *Brain Research Reviews, 31,* 83–104.

Van Oudenhoven, J. P., de Raad, B., Askevis-Leherpeux, F., Boski, P., Brunborg, G. S., Carmona, C., Barelds, D., Hill, C. T., Mlačić, B., Motti, F., Rammstedt, B., & Woods, S. (2008). Terms of abuse as expression and reinforcement of cultures. *International Journal of Intercultural Relations, 32,* 174–185.

Volkan, V., Itzkowitz, N., & Dod, A. W. (1997). *Richard Nixon: A psychobiography.* New York: Columbia University Press.

Vythilingum, B., Stein, D. J., & Soifer, S. (2002). Is 'shy bladder syndrome' a subtype of social anxiety disorders? A survey of people with paruresis. *Depression and Anxiety, 16,* 84–87.

Wahl, C. W., & Golden, J. S. (1963). Psychogenic urinary retention: Report on 6 cases. *Psychosomatic Medicine, 25,* 543–555.

Wales, E., & Brewer, B. (1976). Graffiti in the 1970's. *Journal of Social Psychology, 99,* 115–123.

Walkling, A. (1935). Rupture of the sigmoid by hydrostatic pressure. *Annals of Surgery, 102,* 471–472.

Walsh, J. J. (1912). *Psychotherapy: Including the history of the use of mental influence, directly and indirectly in healing and the principles for the application of energies derived from the mind to the treatment of disease.* New York: Appleton.

Walsh, M., Duffy, J., & Gallagher-Duffy, J. (2007). A more accurate approach to measuring the prevalence of sexual harassment among high school students. *Canadian Journal of Behavioural Science, 39,* 110–118.

Watson, W. L., Bell, J. M., & Wright, L. M. (1992). Osteophytes and marital fights: A single-case clinical research report of chronic pain. *Family Systems Medicine, 10,* 423–435.

Wax, D. E., & Haddox, V. G. (1974). Enuresis, firesetting, and animal cruelty: A useful danger signal in predicting vulnerability of adolescent males to assaultive behavior. *Child Psychiatry and Human Development, 4,* 151–156.

Webster, D. M., & Kruglanski, A. W. (1994). Individual differences in need for closure. *Journal of Personality and Social Psychology, 67,* 1049–1062.

Weil, R. S., Cavanna, A. E., Willoughby, J. M. T., & Robertson, M. M. (2008). Air swallowing as a tic. *Journal of Psychosomatic Research, 65,* 497–500.

Weinberg, M. S., & Williams, C. J. (2005). Fecal matters: Habitus, embodiments, and deviance. *Social Problems, 52,* 315–336.

Wells, J. W. (1989). Sexual language use in different interpersonal contexts: A comparison of gender and sexual orientation. *Archives of Sexual Behavior, 18,* 127–143.

Wheatley, T., & Haidt, J. (2005). Hypnotically induced disgust makes moral judgments more severe. *Psychological Science,* 16, 780–784.

Whitehead, W. E., Palsson, O., & Jones, K. R. (2002). Systematic review of the comorbidity of irritable bowel syndrome with other disorders: What are the causes and implications? *Gastroenterology, 122,* 1140–1156.

Whiting, J. W. M., & Child, I. L. (1953). *Child training and personality: A cross-cultural study.* New Haven and London: Yale University Press.

Whiting, S., & Koller, S. (2007). *Dialogues in solitude: The discursive structures and social functions of male toilet graffiti.* Working paper 126, Centre for the Study of Language in Social Life, Lancaster University.

Whorton, J. C. (2000). *Inner hygiene: Constipation and the pursuit of health in modern society.* Oxford University Press.

Williams, G. E., & Johnson, A. M. (1956). Recurrent urinary retention due to emotional factors: Report of a case. *Psychosomatic Medicine, 18,* 77–80.

Williams, G. W., & Degenhardt, E. T. (1954). Paruresis: A survey of a disorder of micturition. *Journal of General Psychology, 51,* 19–29.

Wise, T. N., & Goldberg, R. L. (1995). Escalation of a fetish: Coprophagia in a nonpsychotic adult of normal intelligence. *Journal of Sex and Marital Therapy, 21,* 272–275.

Witkin, H. A., & Goodenough, D. R. (1981). *Cognitive styles: Essence and origins.* Madison, CT: International Universities Press.

Wober, J. M. (1990). Language and television. In H. Giles & W. P. Robinson (eds), *Handbook of language and social psychology* (pp. 561–582). New York: Wiley.

Wray, M. (2006). *Not quite white: White trash and the boundaries of whiteness.* Durham, NC: Duke University Press.

Yalug, I., Kirmizi-Alsan, E., & Tufan, A. E. (2007). Adult onset pica in the context of anorexia nervosa with major depressive disorder and a history of childhood geophagia: A case report. *Progress in Neuro-psychopharmacology & Biological Psychiatry, 31*, 1341–1342.

Young-Bruehl, E. (1996). *The anatomy of prejudices.* Cambridge, MA: Harvard University Press.

Yovel, I., Revelle, W., & Mineka, S. (2005). Who sees trees before forest? The obsessive-compulsive style of visual attention. *Psychological Science, 16*, 123–129.

Zajonc, R. B., Pietromonaco, P., & Bargh, J. (1982). Independence and interaction of affect and cognition. In M. S. Clark & S. T. Fiske (eds), *Affect and cognition: The 17th annual Carnegie symposium on cognition* (pp. 211–227). Hillsdale, NJ: Erlbaum.

Zeitlin, S. B., & Polivy, J. (1995). Coprophagia as a manifestation of obsessive-compulsive disorder: A case report. *Journal of Behavior Therapy and Experimental Psychiatry, 26*, 57–63.

Zella, S. J., Geenens, D. L., & Horst, J. N. (1998). Repetitive eructation as a manifestation of obsessive-compulsive disorder. *Psychosomatics, 39*, 299–301.

Zhong, C-B., Strejcek, B., & Sivanathan, N. (2010). A clean self can render harsh moral judgment. *Journal of Experimental Social Psychology, 46*, 859–862.

Index